EAT THIS

THIS

WHEN YOU'RE EXPECTING

NOT

THAT!®

Dr. Jennifer Ashton, MD, ABC News Chief Women's Health Correspondent
with **David Zinczenko**, co-founder, Eat This, Not That!

G

GALVANIZED

No book can replace the diagnostic expertise
and medical advice of a trusted physician.
Please be certain to consult with your doctor before
making any decisions that affect your health,
particularly if you suffer from any medical condition or
have any symptom that may require treatment.

Published in the United States by
Galvanized Books,
a division of Galvanized Brands, LLC, New York

Galvanized Books is a trademark of Galvanized Brands, LLC

ISBN 978-0-425-28471-1

Printed in the United States of America on acid-free paper

246897531

Book design by George Karabotsos with Laura White

Cover photograph by Shutterstock. Interior photographs by Thomas MacDonald,
Dan Engongoro, Jeff Harris and Shutterstock.

GALVANIZED

Dedication

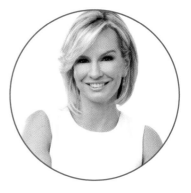

To every woman who's ever worried about what to eat, desired a healthier life, and wondered how much weight to gain—while carrying a person inside them. May this book provide the tools and comfort you need to create your happiest and healthiest self—and child. And to their OB/GYNs and midwives—may this book spark a conversation about how we can make smarter choices for healthier families, in our unified fight against obesity.

—Dr. Jennifer Ashton

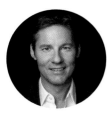

To my mom, and moms everywhere. You taught us the value of a meal made with love.

—David Zinczenko

Acknowledgments

This book is the product of my years of medical training, hundreds of conversations with patients, nutritionists, and industry experts, months of intensive research, and the collective smarts, dedication and raw talent of dozens of individuals. My undying thanks to those who have helped to make this book a possibility:

David Zinczenko, the co-founder of Eat This, Not That!, and his team at Galvanized, an extraordinary collection of men and women who have come together to create a business, establish an empire, and change the way a media company thinks. Your hard work and dedication is an inspiration.

The team at Fit Pregnancy, who provided the delicious recipes and other content (with a special shout-out to former Fit Preggers Peg Moline and Andrea Bartz), and Dana Points at Parents, for her invaluable insights.

Kim Hekimian, PhD, and Sharon Akabas, PhD—my course directors and professors at Columbia University's Institute of Human Nutrition.

The folks at Penguin Random House, in particular Marnie Cochran, Gina Centrello, Kim Hovey, Richard Callison and Bill Takes.

Barbara Fedida, Robin Roberts, George Stephanopoulos, Lara Spencer, Amy Robach, Ginger Zee, Patty Neger, Simone Swink, Alberto Orso, Greg Tufaro and the best team ever at *Good Morning America*.

Jay McGraw, Dr. Travis Stork, Patty Ciano and Jeff Hudson and the brilliant minds at *The Doctors*.

Andy McNicol, Jennifer Rudolph Walsh and my awesome WME team. And to the best family ever, without whom this book wouldn't exist.

—Dr. Jennifer Ashton

Contents

"Should I cook my deli meat?" Very good question—don't miss page 144.

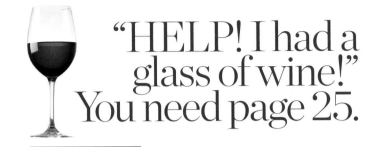

"HELP! I had a glass of wine!" You need page 25.

"I'm craving ice cream! Which brand is best?" Pick any from page 262.

"IS THERE A FOOD THAT WILL MAKE MY BABY SMART?" YES! SEE PAGE 85.

"Do I have to give up diet soda? For real?" Well ... see page 24.

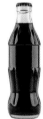

"How much weight should I gain?" Depends—see page 38.

"Will probiotics help with my bloat?" Find out on page 18.

"What kinds of cheese are OK to eat?" Those on page 222.

Contents

Congratulations!

By getting this book, you've taken control of your weight, your health, your wallet, your food supply—and, most importantly, your baby's future. That kicking you'll soon feel is actually her trying to high-five you: Best Mom Ever.

Why? For the past decade, *Eat This, Not That!* has been America's #1 resource for what to eat for your healthiest and happiest life. *Expecting* is designed to be that for you *and* the next generation—the one in your belly. That's why we couldn't be happier to introduce not just the best person to write it, but the only doctor who could: Dr. Jennifer Ashton, OB/GYN. When not on TV—as Chief Women's Health Correspondent at ABC News and co-host of *The Doctors*—Dr. Ashton runs a thriving full-time OB/GYN practice, and is the country's only doctor who is newly Board-certified in Obesity Medicine, and getting a Master's Degree in Nutrition at Columbia University.

She believes food can be medicine, if you eat the right food. It's a mission that's perfectly aligned with ours.

Eating for a Healthy Baby

There is simply no greater single way to foster a healthy baby than by the foods you eat. Studies show that a balanced diet—like the one detailed in *Eat This, Not That! When You're Expecting*—leads to fewer complications, easier deliveries, fewer defects, and happier, fitter babies after they're born. (Yup, what you consume today can dictate what they want to eat tomorrow—and how often they get sick.)

Without this book, it'd be impossible to know which brands to buy, which restaurants to trust, and how to cook at home. Making the right food choice—in a world of health halos, hidden sugars, and deceptive marketing—is hard even when you're not pregnant.

You'd think it would be easier. When the first *Eat This, Not That!* was released, there was no way to know how many calories were sandwiched into your Subway sandwich, how much fat and salt a Denny's Grand Slam slams you with, or how much totally unnatural sugar, hydrogenated oil, and preservatives were in Wendy's "Natural-Cut" Fries. The ingredients—even the number of calories—in the foods Americans ate every day remained one of the great mysteries.

But in those ensuing years, everything about the way we eat has changed. Today, thanks to the outcry unleashed by *Eat This, Not That!*, most restaurants now post their calorie counts, and share ingredients, too.

Unfortunately, Americans don't know what to do with all that information—and can't tell what's true.

Check, Please

In a 2014 study in the journal *Public Health Nutrition*, people were asked to report their food intake over the course of 48 hours. Those who ate at a restaurant during that time took in an average of 200 calories per day more than those who prepared all of their own meals.

(Those who ate in sit-down restaurants actually consumed slightly more calories than those who ordered from fast food joints.) It takes 3,500 calories to create a pound of body weight; so according to that study, our eat-in, take-out, culture is adding just under 21 pounds of extra fat to our bodies every year.

Or more. In less than five years, the percentage of our calories that come from food outside the home has risen to 43 percent—the highest since the USDA began tracking such statistics. That means we're cooking less and less each year.

With studies showing how weight gain and obesity can lead to troubled pregnancies, you can see why the time for *Eat This, Not That! When You're Expecting* is now. Understanding what's in our food is harder than ever. And *Eat This, Not That!* is going to be working harder than ever to keep you informed.

Dr. Ashton will see you now.

—David Zinczenko
Founder, Eat This, Not That!

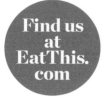

Introd

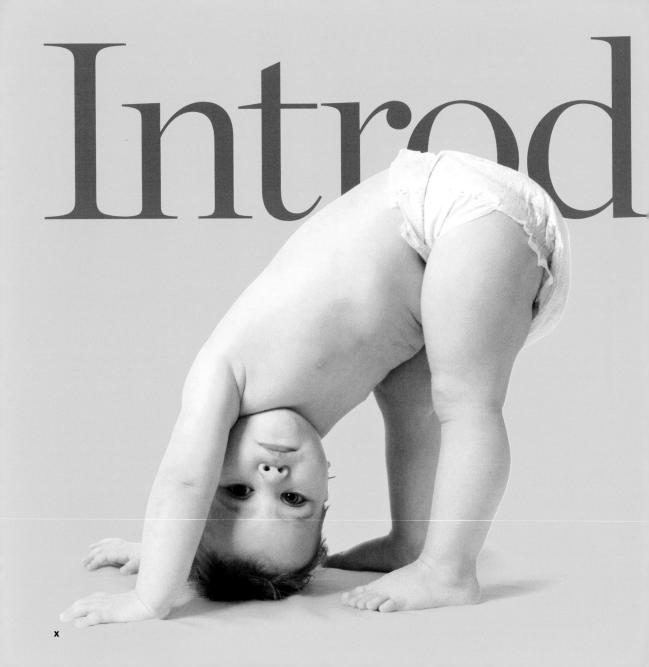

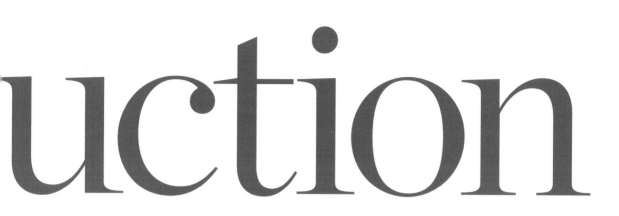

uction

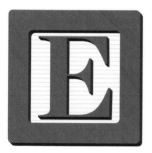

EVERYONE SAYS, when you're pregnant, you're eating for two. But I wrote this book because I want to change that thinking. I want you to eat for *you*.

What do I mean by that? My patients know. As an OB/GYN with a full-time practice—not to mention in my roles as Chief Women's Health Correspondent at ABC News, and as co-host of *The Doctors*—it's my mission to deliver the most accessible, up-to-date and action-able information to ensure you stay healthy during your pregnancy, and deliver a beautiful, bouncy bundle of joy at the end. (And I've delivered more than 1,500 of them!)

That means you'll need to know the essential vitamins and key nutrients your little one needs to grow, and which foods stave off defects, gestational diabetes, and other complications. And it means you should ask your OB/GYN or midwife to join you in learning, so you can work together to control your nutri-tion. With 66% of reproductive-age women overweight or obese, the need to combat unhealthy and uninformed eating is a responsibility we all share.

But "eating for you" also means being practical.

Because I know you're more than just a mom-to-be. You're a mom-to-be who's got a thousand other jobs, from career woman to budding chef to amateur yogi to professional Pinsta-grammer and possibly, maybe, if you have 5 minutes left, wife (and perhaps you're a mom already, in which case, you know what I mean). No matter how you spend your time, chances are you don't have much of it—and certainly don't want to spend the next nine months measuring the folate counts in every box of cereal, or starving on your next road trip because Burger King doesn't serve kale.

You need nutrition. And you need it now. And although cooking your own food is the surest way to maintain a healthy diet, you probably can't do so every day for the next nine months.

That's why I wrote *Eat This, Not That! When You're Expecting*, the only book of its kind by a doctor qualified to talk about nutrition, physiology, and disease—who will also tell you what to do the next time you're at the salad bar, in the yogurt aisle, or at Mickey D's.

Because, let's be honest, momma's gonna crave a little Mickey D's.

And she's going to need clean energy, too. That's why I'll also tell you how delicious wild salmon, fresh and creamy smoothies, and time-saving foods like rotisserie chicken or frozen meals can be essential building blocks for healthy trimesters. In the end, you'll discover not just *what* to eat, but how to enjoy the foods you love.

You'll eat for you, while nourishing baby, too.

Why We Need This Book—Now

If you were to walk into my office, the first thing you'd realize about me is, I'm a woman (what gave it away?), a doctor (with an M.D. from Columbia), and a mother (on my desk are photos of my two kids, now teenagers somehow).

But shortly after that, you'd learn I'm also formally educated in Nutrition. Oddly enough, not too many people can say they're all of those things.

During my 16 years of practicing medicine, I've met a lot of nutritionists who aren't credentialed doctors and a lot of doctors who aren't credentialed nutritionists. That's why, after becoming an M.D., I decided to get Board Certified in obesity medicine, and complete a Master's in Human Clinical Nutrition at Columbia. I needed those credentials to talk about nutrition because I talk about nutrition *a lot*, and not just with my patients. When you're on TV, telling women to lose weight, gain weight (in a healthy way), and eat right, you better know what you're talking about. More importantly, you better also provide actionable advice.

It's amazing how few doctors, even OB/GYNs, do that. They don't because they can't.

When I went to medical school at Columbia, and graduated in 2000, we had almost zero formal nutritional training. Over the last 15 years, we've seen a growing shift in not just interest in nutrition but in nutritional information. The medical community is finally catching up, realizing food is medicine.

Thanks to *Eat This, Not That!*, consumers have wised up, too, and demand to know what's in their meals. If food is medicine, this book tells you which to take.

How to Eat Right Every Time

Pregnancy, labor, and delivery are athletic events, so why not train for them? Nutrition is a key part of that training, and as a result, can be daunting. I encourage my patients not to associate pregnancy with the "d-word." For some, it's "disease"—no judgment; it can feel that way on dark days. For others, it's a word that can be even more loaded: "diet." But we should not look at the next nine months as being filled with limitations; we should look at them as an opportunity. Here's a few thoughts to remember:

It's never too late to change

… or tweak or improve the way you eat, and that goes for everyone. I've met women for whom finding themselves pregnant is the catalyst they need to finally start eating healthier. "I don't care if I've been poisoning myself," some have told me, "but I don't wanna poison someone else!" It's their lightbulb moment. I've also met hardcore dieters who actually have to take in *more* calories, which is a shock to them. When I was getting my Master's, we had to analyze our own eating and do a three-day food diary. I went into it thinking, "No way can I eat better!" And then I found I was 30% deficient in micronutrients. It's not like I was eating fast food drive-through every day; I just wasn't getting a wide variety of fruits and veg.

My point is, everyone can improve something—and it's never too late.

It's not about how you look

We live in a vain and superficial culture, and the headlines prove it: "Blast that Baby Weight." "20 Post-Baby Slimdowns Secrets." "How Beyoncé Lost the Belly!" As if somehow you should go through this process and never look like you've grown another human being!

The silver lining—and I always try to find one—is that at least we're talking about the importance of maternal weight gain. In the past—as late as 30 years ago—there was almost no attention paid to it during pregnancy. But that's not healthy for the mom or the baby. So I try to bring it back to a happy medium. You could use pregnancy to get into the greatest shape of your

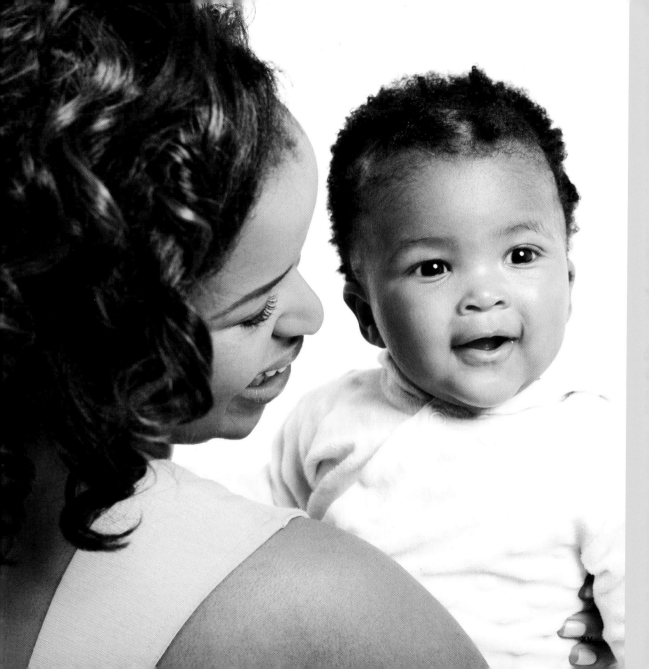

life. Or you could continue your current fitness routine, and just eat the foods in this book. Do it because it feels good; the looks will come.

It's not about making a mistake

Wine, sushi, carbs—so many moms think, "If I do one thing wrong, I'll ruin my baby for life." But honestly, if pregnancies were so precarious, we wouldn't have a civilization. Take control over what you can control. For example, you shouldn't eat certain fish when pregnant, because they're high in mercury. But consider the dose and frequency. If you slip up and eat shark in a fish gumbo, there's only a very, very small chance anything will go wrong. That doesn't mean you should eat more shark; it just means you should absorb the rules in this book and worry less. Pace yourself. As a mom, I know the worries don't end when the placenta comes out.

How to Use This Book

At its core, *Eat This, Not That! When You're Expecting* is meant to tell you what to eat when you're pregnant.

You'll learn:

- **The essential nutrients, and where to find them**
- **What to order when you're eating out**
- **What to buy, aisle-by-aisle in the supermarket**
- **How to cook delicious craving crushers and healthy meals**
- **And how to stop worrying, live healthfully, and enjoy the next amazing nine months.**

But the reason it's so distinctive is that it's practical. I offer delicious recipes, compliments of Fit Pregnancy, but also tell you what to eat at the drive-through, or during a burger craving, or when you want ice cream—so you can buy the right kind for you, and ask yourself: If a food is not a good fuel for my body, and my baby, why eat it?

So I Can Eat Ice Cream?

The burning question—right? Of course you can eat ice cream, and I'll tell you why in a moment. But first, I want to say that I'm not a big fan of labeling any food "bad" or "good." In medicine, few things are that simple.

Ice cream is no different. In fact, I'd give it an A: it has calcium, protein, fat. (Find my favorites on page 262.) It's only problematic when we eat too

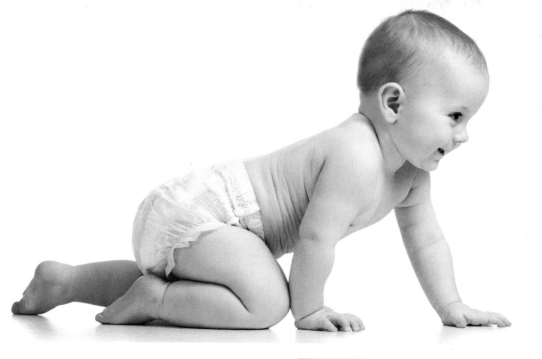

much, or add too many toppings. That's why I think *Eat This, Not That! When You're Expecting* is the perfect title. It's not meant to be the definitive bible. It's meant to show you a better way to eat.

And if you're feeling nauseous, or having trouble gaining weight, or, heck, just want a nice dessert after a long day—eat ice cream! Stop by my office. I'll write you a prescription.

To your health—and baby's, too,
Dr. Jennifer Ashton,
Board-Certified OB/GYN

My Thanks to Fit Pregnancy

This book would not have been possible without the editorial team at Fit Pregnancy, who graciously provided delicious recipes, engaging copy, and other valuable information for *Eat This, Not That! When You're Expecting*. The brand recently relaunched in a major way, and is necessary reading for pregnant women—check it out at fitpregnancy.com.

Chapter

1

What to Eat for Your Baby —and You

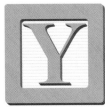

YOUR BODY IS A MIRACLE—and right now, it's about to create one.

For the last few decades, it's allowed you to walk, laugh, cry, downward-dog, and dance all night. Right now, it's embarking on possibly its most incredible feat yet: Building a tiny human inside of you.

To keep it humming, this glorious machine of yours needs certain nutrients—substances it pulls out of the food you eat—to help you look good and feel great. And for most of your life, your body has been able to fake its way through; a salad here and a serving of chicken breast there has made up for game-day indulgences, Twizzler-fueled movie nights, and more than a few ladies' nights out.

But when you're pregnant, it's hard not to worry 24/7 about whether you're eating the right things, eating enough of them, or doing something wrong at snacktime. The Truth? There's nothing wrong with spending some quality time with your buddies Ben and Jerry when the craving arises (and it probably will). All that really matters is that most of the time, you're eating healthy stuff—and that you're getting a daily flow of certain key nutrients—compounds that are critical for your baby's development. It's really not rocket science!

Some might finger wag and tell you you're now the personal chef and nutritionist for your babe-to-be—because you do have complete control over what nutrients baby's getting—but I know you're so much more than just a glorified baby carrier. You're a smart, strong, energetic woman who also wants to continue leading the full and fun life you always have. Eating right won't just set the stage for a healthy life for your child, it will also ensure that you can be as active and vibrant as ever when you enter this exciting and magical new chapter of your life.

That's why *Eat This, Not That! When You're Expecting* is all about making these wise choices without a second thought. With a series of simple swaps, and a focus on the right nutrients, you can:

Help Your Child Be Fit, Not Chubby

Of course the number one concern of every mother-to-be is that her child will be healthy and happy—no matter what size, shape, or crazy taste in music she may turn out to have! But I'm sure we'd all prefer to think our children could avoid physically and emotionally difficult weight battles later on. The truth is, how you eat now can actually help your tiny one's chances of having and maintaining a healthy weight later in life. Researchers writing in the *International Journal of Obesity* in 2014 found that what a

mother ate while pregnant, as well as how stressed she was, can affect baby's genetic propensity for obesity. And while completely stress-free pregnancies might be the stuff of fairy tales, the information in this book will make smart nutritional decisions one less thing you need to worry about.

Boost Baby's Ivy League Chances

Already thinking about Junior's college education? You're not the only mom-to-be to be about thirty steps ahead! The great news is that studies have shown that a healthy diet during pregnancy can boost your baby's brain power. One found that children whose mothers took supplements of cod liver oil during pregnancy and lactation scored higher on academic tests at age 4 than children of moms who had taken corn oil supplements.

(The magic nutrient was omega-3 fatty acids, which you'll read about in this chapter.) Other studies found that children of women with the lowest percentage of iodine in their bloodstreams were in the lowest quartile for verbal IQ, reading accuracy and reading comprehension. (To make sure you're getting enough iodine, toss the artisanal sea salt and use standard, iodine-fortified table salt—sparingly—when you're flavoring your meals.)

Let Your Little One Breathe Easier

Babies are less likely to develop autoimmune issues like allergies and asthma if they are exposed to a nutrient-rich diet while in the womb, according to a report from the Academy of Nutrition and Dietetics.

Set the stage for healthy habits. Crazy but true: Eating a smart diet of healthy meals and snacks can alter your child's brain development, programming her preference for nutritious fruits, veggies, and grains later in life!

Step Up Baby's Social Game

At least in animal studies, researchers have found that the offspring of moms who eat a diet rich in choline, a nutrient found in eggs and other lean proteins—easy to get once you know what you're looking for!—are less likely to suffer from social behavior deficits and anxiety. Other studies show that proper nutrition can give a child better ability to control her behavior. That could mean fewer tantrums for you to deal with, and more happy, lifelong friendships in her future.

Protect Your Child from Premature Birth

Moms-to-be who eat a diet rich in fruits, veggies, lean meats, and whole grains are 15 percent more likely to carry their child to term than women who lean toward sugar, fat, and processed foods, according to research from Sahlgrenska Academy University of Gothenberg in Sweden.

Help Yourself Have an Easier Labor and Delivery

Women with normal to high levels of vitamin D needed fewer pain meds during delivery than those with a deficiency, according to research presented at the American Society of Anesthesiologists' annual conference. The study's authors speculate that the vitamin is linked to stronger muscle contractions, which make labor quicker and easier. Amen to that!

THAT'S A LOT OF PAYOFF just from switching your nightly snack from Hot Pockets to something fresh and healthy. Despite all the evidence that great nutrition is key—and how simple it can be to eat right—a large study published in the journal *Public Health Nutrition* found that 80 percent of American women of childbearing age don't get enough vitamin A, 78 percent aren't taking in enough vitamin D, and 92 percent aren't getting enough fiber. A separate report from the Centers for Disease Control showed that 16 million American women are at risk of iron deficiency. That's why we're here to make breakfast a breeze, snacking simple, and meals *more* than manageable.

In chapter two, we've outlined a healthy, balanced, and most of all easy-to-follow diet that will not only see you through your first trimester, but serve as a great eating plan while you're nursing, when you're ready to lose the baby weight, and throughout the rest of your life. It's a plan that centers on five crucial supernutrients: calcium, iron, folic acid, vitamin D, and omega-3 fatty acids. You'll soon see just how simple (and satisfying!) it can be to pack them into even the busiest of days.

THE **EAT THIS, NOT THAT!** SUPER

CALCIUM The Bone Builder!

So much of your tiny bundle's body—his bones and teeth, muscles, and nerves—depend on calcium as a major building block. And getting plenty of this element protects your own skeleton, too. Unfortunate but true, your body's so eager to knit together strong bones in your baby, that if you don't get enough of the nutrient, it could pull calcium out of your own bone system, leaving you at risk of fractures. Not such a good look. Try to get need 1,000 mg a day.

So where can you find all the calcium you'll need during your pregnancy? Cheese and yogurt are obvious sources, but you'll also find calcium in fortified cereal, leafy greens, tofu, sardines, and bone-in salmon.

⟳ *Drink This*

Almond milk and 1% milk. If you're a die-hard dairy queen, stick with 1% pasteurized milk. Drinking more than eight ounces of whole milk a day is linked with larger-than-normal birth weight, research suggests. And the unpasteurized stuff (say, from the farmers' market) could contain bacteria such as *Listeria*—which could jeopardize your entire pregnancy. Meanwhile, unsweetened almond milk provides dairy milk's calcium with fewer calories.

⟳ *Eat This*

Collard greens and other sautéed greens. A cooked cup of the Southern favorite contains 268 mg of calcium, plus loads of healthy vitamin A. Other dark, leafy greens are even more calcium packed—try watercress, curly kale, and dandelion greens.

Sardines. Each little fish contains 46 mg of calcium—so just four gets you almost 20 percent of the way toward your daily goal.

⟳ *Other Key Sources*

Yogurt	Figs	Oranges
Cottage cheese	Broccoli	Kelp
Eggs	Broccoli rabe	White beans
Sunflower seeds	Sweet potatoes	

⟳ *Not That*

Calcium chews. A large review of studies published in the *British Medical Journal* suggests that calcium supplements—but not calcium in food—may increase heart attack risk when taken long-term. Talk to your doctor before going on daily high-dose calcium supplements.

NUTRIENT CHECKLIST

*Fully cook raw meat and fish

IRON The Blood Maker!

Never thought you'd be a body builder? Think again! Body building is literally what you're doing as you're creating a new life during pregnancy, which means you've got to be pumping that iron—at least in nutrient form. During pregnancy, you need 27 mg of iron a day—about twice as much as you did before you became pregnant. The reason? Extra iron helps your body make more blood, which helps shuttle the needed amounts of oxygen to your baby. Being low in the mineral ups the risk of premature birth, low birth weight, and even maternal and infant mortality.

Your system is happiest getting iron from animal protein, and cooked red meat, turkey, sardines, and chicken are great sources. You'll also find it in spinach, beans, nuts, prunes, and peas, although your body has to work a bit harder to metabolize the iron in plant-based sources.

⟲ Eat This

Grass-fed lean beef—ground. Three ounces of the stuff (think the size of a deck of cards) provides 3.2 mg of digestible iron. Just cook it thoroughly so there's no trace of pink or blood—now is not the time to risk getting sick from a parasite.

Dark chocolate. No joke! When it comes to iron, ounce for ounce, your favorite indulgence makes lean beef chuck look like a lightweight. Just one ounce of the stuff with 70–85 percent cacao provides 3.4 mg of your daily 27 mg goal.

Pumpkin seeds. The great thing about these crunchy seeds is that you only need to consume them in small quantities to reap the health benefits. One ounce contains more than eight grams of protein and is also high in iron, potassium, phosphorus, magnesium and zinc (important for a healthy immune system).

Add into salads, oats, and yogurt, or pop them in your mouth as-is for a quick snack.

⟲ Other Key Sources

Nettle tea

Spinach and collard greens

Broccoli rabe

Iron-fortified cereal or oatmeal

Lentils

Kidney beans

Chickpeas

Pumpkin seeds

Clam chowder or well-cooked clams

Chicken

⟲ Not That

Beef or chicken liver It contains a huge concentration of easy-to-break-down iron—more than 3.5 mg per serving—so you may see it on lists of what to eat to up your iron intake. But because having too much vitamin A can harm your baby—and this stuff has a lot of it!—you'll want to steer clear until after baby's born.

Your body absorbs iron best when you eat it with vitamin C-rich foods, like citrus!

FOLIC ACID aka Folate, the Safeguarder!

You've probably been hearing about folic acid since you first learned you were pregnant—but trust us on this, its importance isn't being overhyped. This pregnancy superstar, also called folate, is a B vitamin that is crucial in protecting against debilitating defects in baby's brain and spine called neural tube defects. Additionally, a study at Duke University found that folate can make developing fetuses more resistant to the dangers of bisphenol-A (BPA), an all-too-common plastic-based chemical that scientists are now linking to obesity. Folic acid should definitely be part of your prenatal vitamin's all-star lineup, but your body can absorb it best through the food you eat, so be sure to get some that way, too.

You need 600 mcg a day. The best sources—those that provide at least 20 percent of your daily value per serving—to keep in your fridge include: romaine lettuce, spinach, kale, endive, collard greens, and Swiss chard. Other sources include Brussels sprouts, avocado, and peas.

⏻ Eat This

Cooked lentils. A cup of filling lentils contains 358 mcg of folate—more than half your pregnancy RDA—and just a gram of fat. Cooked pinto beans, black eyed peas, chickpeas, and kidney beans (basically, anything that'd be good in a bowl of veggie chili) also score well for their folate content.

Cooked spinach. Heating up the veggie concentrates its nutrients, so a cup contains 263 mcg of folic acid—four times as much as the raw stuff.

⏻ Other Key Sources

Okra	Avocado
Tangerines	Tomato juice
Asparagus	Cantaloupe
Kidney beans	Enriched pasta
Broccoli	Eggs
Sunflower seeds	

⏻ Not That

Sprouted lentils. Sounds so healthy, right? But a raw veggie swimming in its own vat of water can harbor harmful bacteria, like *salmonella*, *E. coli*, and *listeria*, which can threaten the life of your child. Avoid raw bean sprouts and other sprouted veggies for the same reason.

No time to cook? Pour a bowl of Kellogg's All Bran! It's high in folate.

VITAMIN D The Skin Developer!

The vitamin is a bit of a wonder nutrient: It works hand-in-hand with calcium to help baby's bones and teeth develop, and it's key for healthy skin and eyesight (yours and your bundle's). Plus, it may be associated with a lower chance of preeclampsia—a serious condition that can threaten your health. We all know our bodies produce vitamin D when sunshine hits our skin, but given skin cancer risks (not to mention the fact that premature aging and pregnancy-related dark spots aren't so cute), your best bet is to get your D through yummy snacks and meals. Great food sources include D-fortified dairy and fatty fish such as salmon.

So how much do you need? All women, including those who are pregnant, need 600 international units (IU) of vitamin D per day. Talk to your doctor before taking any supplements, but most experts agree that when you have a deficiency (a blood test will reveal this), taking an additional 1,000 to 2,000 IU per day in pill form is safe during pregnancy.

Eat This

Grilled, baked, or roasted wild salmon. The tasty fish is one of nature's best sources of D, with a three-ounce serving packing 447 IU (that takes care of most of your daily 600 IU right there). Make sure to cook it to at least 145 degrees Fahrenheit—all fish and meat should be eaten piping hot.

Fortified cereal. It's perhaps the easiest way to get this sometimes elusive nutrient. Look for whole-grain options that contain at least 40 IU of vitamin D, without artificial colors or loads of sugar, and pair with a half-cup of fortified skim milk, and you've taken in 100 IU in one fell swoop.

Other Key Sources

Pork loin

Eggs

Shiitake mushrooms

Fortified cow's milk

Wild mackerel

Fish oil

Atlantic herring
(very low in mercury)

Yogurt

Sardines

Not That

Seared tuna. Its D content is respectable at best (70 IU in a half-ounce fillet), but the bigger problem is the preparation. Under-cooked fish may contain parasites or bacteria; that's why you're steering clear of your favorite sushi joint for nine months. Remember that raw-in-the-middle fish (and meat!) are off-limits till D-day.

Look for milk labeled "fortified" or "Vitamin D."

OMEGA-3s The Smart Maker!

Omega-3 fatty acids—specifically eicosapentaeonic acid, aka EPA, and docosahexaenoic acid, aka DHA (don't worry, we're not going to quiz you on the crazy scientific names!)—have a whole host of roles to play when it comes to baby's development. In addition to helping build your little one's brain and eyes, they can also lower your babe's chances of suffering from asthma and allergies, prevent pre-term birth, help you fight off depression during and after your pregnancy, and reduce your risk of heart disease. Still not convinced? Experts from the National Institutes of Health have found that moms who eat several weekly servings of fatty fish give birth to children with IQs five points higher than the children of their fish-averse peers. Try to get 200 mg a day.

Obviously, Omega-3s are awesome, but how much of them do you need in your diet? As of 2014, the FDA recommends pregnant women eat 8 to 12 ounces of fish or shellfish—that's about three servings—per week. Yep, these long-chain fatty acids are plenty important.

If you're shunning swimmers from a fear of mercury, know that fish are your friends during pregnancy, and that your risk of mercury poisoning is nearly non-existent if you're smart about what you eat: Substantial levels of mercury build up only in large sea creatures that eat plenty of other sea creatures—think carnivores like sharks and swordfish.

Eat This

Cod, Halibut, Pollock, and Wild Salmon. All are solid sources of the omega-3s you and your baby need—plus they're low in mercury, making them super pregnancy-friendly.

Light Canned Tuna. Thanks to its low levels of contaminants, light canned tuna also gets the thumbs-up; experts suggest enjoying one 6-ounce serving (that's a typical can) up to six times a month.

Other Key Sources

Wild rice

Red lentils

Chia seeds

Ground mustard

Spinach

Winter squash

Fontina cheese (okay because it is pasteurized)

Walnuts

Flax seeds

Not That

Swordfish. Sure, it's rich in omega-3s, and it's a vitamin D powerhouse, with a 3-ounce steak containing 566 IU of the nutrient. But because of its high mercury content, it's not safe for pregnant women. Other mercurial baddies: tilefish, shark, and king mackerel.

For "The Fish-Hater's Guide to Omega-3s," turn to page 70.

THE **EAT THIS, NOT THAT!**
OTHER KEY NUTRIENTS

Vitamin C

You know that C is the go-to vitamin whenever someone in your social orbit is getting sick; its role in bolstering the immune system is well-established. But in pregnancy, C plays another critical role: It helps your body absorb iron. That's important, because your body uses iron to make new blood cells for you and your baby, to fill those extra miles of vessels, arteries and capillaries the two of you will be sharing. And by ensuring that you're absorbing iron from your food, C will also help keep you from becoming tired or irritable. You'll find vitamin C exactly where you'd expect: in citrus, as well as kiwi, mangoes, strawberries, broccoli, and peppers.

Potassium

Potassium sits on the other side of your body's seesaw from sodium, doing its best to keep that big salty monster from causing havoc with your blood pressure. When potassium drops, blood pressure can rise, and you can also experience swelling and leg cramps. By eating potassium-rich foods like bananas, sweet potatoes, yogurt, and beans, you're keeping your body's fluids and electrolytes in balance. Potassium helps your body build muscles, and keeps your muscles and nerves in close communication, so when you hear, "It's time to push," your body will be primed for maximum athletic performance.

Protein

Proteins are the building blocks of your baby. From skin and bone to blood, muscle, heart and (maybe) a little tuft of hair, proteins fit together like Legos to create the amazing little form inside of you. They're also what helps your body grow and repair itself, as well, whether you're laying down new rivers of blood vessels or storing milk in your breasts. You'll find "complete" proteins—meaning forms that are ready to be converted right into body tissue—in all animal and dairy products, and your body knows how to cobble incomplete proteins, from sources like whole grains, nuts, beans, and even vegetables, into the muscle-making protein it needs.

Magnesium

Magnesium is the traffic-control mineral of your body. At any given time, it's helping to direct any number of the more than 300 enzymes in your body that help regulate metabolism, protein formation, and muscle contractions, among other things. And by helping to transport calcium and potassium across cell membranes, magnesium helps maintain normal heart rhythms and proper blood pressure. That's critical, because a magnesium deficiency can put you at risk for muscle cramps and preeclampsia. You'll find magnesium in dark-green leafy vegetables, nuts, and fortified breakfast cereals.

Vitamin B6

Vitamin B6 is a critical brain builder. It helps the body build and repair tissues in the nervous system, and helps in the manufacture of hormones like serotonin (the "feel good" hormone) and melatonin, which helps regulate your body's clock. It also helps in maintaining the soft tissues of the digestive and muscular systems. Because it plays such a role in stabilizing the brain and the belly, doctors will often use it to treat nausea and vomiting during pregnancy. You'll find it in abundance in chickpeas, fatty fish like tuna and salmon, and fortified breakfast cereals.

Zinc

Although it's a mineral, zinc is very similar to vitamin C in two important ways: First, your body can't make it or store it, so you need to ensure you're getting zinc from your diet regularly. And second, it plays a major role in protecting you from colds and flus, so this already uncomfortable time at least passes without any additional health woes. Zinc helps support the growth of your baby by aiding in the synthesis of protein and DNA. You'll find zinc in fortified breakfast cereals, as well as seafood and beef.

Vitamin B12

Like other B vitamins, B12 is an essential part of a healthy nervous system. B12 deficiency is rare because it's found in most animal products, but when it occurs it can put baby at risk for developmental disorders. It comes from meat, poultry, fish, eggs, and dairy, but you can also get it in some fortified cereals and soy milk. If you're a vegan, you'll need to take a B12 supplement every day.

THE IMPORTANCE OF A HEALTHY MICROBIOME

Microbiome. It sounds like an exciting new addition to EPCOT Center, or the title of the next big space-age thriller. What it is, in reality, is a crazy United Nations of bacteria—some of which are awesome and others . . . well, not so much.

These diverse bacteria battle it out inside your stomach every day. The prize: control over the mechanisms that regulate your hormones and help determine how you metabolize food, react to stress, and store fat. And more and more research is showing that when the good guys win, both you and your babe-to-be benefit. A report in *Pediatric Research* suggests that a healthy microbiome can protect both you and your little one against immune-system flare-ups like allergies, while a study out of The University of Queensland in Australia hints that it may also help you avoid preeclampsia, gestational diabetes, vaginal infections, and excess weight gain.

Likewise, there are some pretty serious consequences if not-so-great bacteria is allowed to run amok in your system.

One study, published in the journal *Pediatric Research*, noted that an out-of-whack microbiome during pregnancy may impair the baby's brain development and could even lead to life-long neurological issues. Another study (from McMaster University in Canada) suggests that a mom-to-be's unhealthy microbiome predisposes her offspring to obesity.

The obvious conclusion: You want the good guys to come out on top. Here's how to make it happen:

GET MORE FIBER

It's a *prebiotic*—one step ahead of probiotics. Good bacteria love it, and when you feed them their favorite food, they flourish, crowding out the bad bacteria. Aim to nosh on lots of roughage and whole grains.

AVOID SUGARY, FATTY FOODS

Yes, you crave them. You know who else does? The havoc-wreaking bad bacteria that want to take over your gut. Encourage the good guys to win with

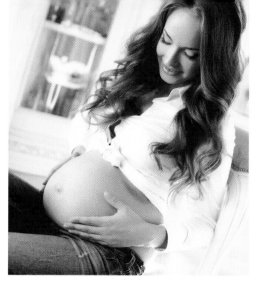

a healthy diet based on fresh fruits, veggies, whole grains, and lean protein—not processed foods.

EAT YOGURT AND FERMENTED FOODS

Kimchi, kefir, and miso contain good-for-you bacteria, in addition to yogurt. Talk to your doctor before reaching for anything unpasteurized—for example, kombucha teas. The same process that breeds the good stuff could leave you vulnerable to pregnancy-threatening bacterial infections.

MINIMIZE UNNECESSARY ANTIBIOTIC USE

Antibiotics kill off bacteria good and bad, leaving your gut with a sad, non-diverse crop of survivors. No bueno.

NEWS FLASH
You're Not Actually "Eating for Two"

Yes, you're the sole supplier of nutrients to your own body as well as that of your growing baby, but that doesn't mean your caloric needs have doubled. In fact, eating way more than you usually would will just lead to excess weight gain, potentially longer and more complicated labor, pregnancy-induced hypertension, and gestational diabetes—all things that can put your health, and that of your unborn child, at risk.

In short: Having a passenger along for the ride doesn't mean you need extra trips to the fueling station. During your first trimester, you should be following a healthy, sensible eating plan that any woman, pregnant or not, could follow. In your second trimester, you'll add a mere 300 calories (that's as simple as having an extra container of yogurt, a handful of nuts, and an apple). And in your third trimester, you'll add 150 calories more. Our trimester-by-trimester eating plan starts on page 31. Easy. Peasy.

PRENATAL VITAMINS A–Z

Even the healthiest eater might need to fill some gaps to give her baby all the nutrients she needs to grow. Here's what you should know about prenatal vitamins.

Start Early

If you can, begin taking a good prenatal multivitamin three months before you start trying to get pregnant. That's because the egg starts maturing about three months before it is released, so it's critical that the nutrients be in your system. Especially important is folic acid, so start taking an over-the-counter supplement with 600 mg even before you start trying to conceive.

Make Sure You Get the Big Three

The three most important nutrients are folic acid, iron, and calcium. Folic acid (the synthetic form of folate, which is more easily absorbed) has been shown to cut the incidence of neural tube defects, such as spina bifida, in half, and is vital for the production of new and healthy red blood cells. On top of that, it may prevent certain cancers and heart disease. Iron is important for the delivery of oxygen to the baby and prevents anemia in the mom; and calcium helps build your baby's bones without taking calcium from yours.

Take With Food

And if you are experiencing morning (or all-day) sickness, take before bed with a small glass of milk.

Think About Supplementing

If your multivitamin doesn't have at least 1,000 milligrams of calcium, you might need a supplement. And most prenatals don't give you the recommended daily 200 milligrams of DHA; you can get adequate amounts from a fish oil capsule, which is safe and mercury free.

Know Your Multi

Even though prescription prenatal vitamins are regulated by the federal Food and Drug Administration (FDA), they are not required to contain all recommended nutrients at all recommended levels. Check out our prenatal vitamin picks below, and then work with your OB to find one that fulfills your requirements.

SOME SMART CHOICES

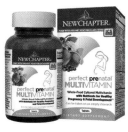

New Chapter Perfect Prenatal Multivitamin contains probiotics, minerals, and organic, whole-food vitamins.

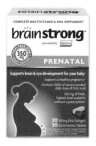

Brainstrong Prenatal vitamins include a vegetarian DHA supplement.

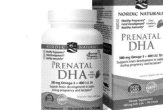

Nordic Naturals Prenatal DHA provides more than double the recommended amount of omega-3s (450 milligrams) in one dose.

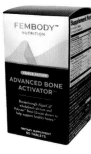

Fembody Nutrition Advanced Bone Activator contains vitamin D and 750 milligrams of organic, plant-based calcium.

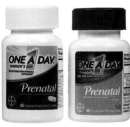

One a Day Women's Prenatal delivers pregnancy nutrients in a multivitamin and a DHA supplement.

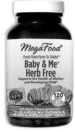

Megafood Baby and Me Herb Free is vegetarian and gluten- and soy-free.

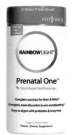

Rainbow Light Prenatal One Multivitamin is vegan and wheat-, gluten-, and sugar-free.

Just Don't Eat These Foods!

You've already got enough to stress about: Which family member will hate your absolute favorite baby name? Which stroller will navigate your neighborhood best? If Prince William had so much trouble figuring out the car seat, how the heck are you supposed to figure this thing out? And, perhaps most worrying of all, how much will a 4-year college cost 18 years from now?

Since stress can have such a negative impact on your health and the health of your child, we're going to make eating wisely super-simple for you, with this list of red-light foods from the U.S. Department of Health & Human Services. Steer clear of these baddies and you'll feel good knowing you're treating your babe (and yourself!) to nutrients from only the safest sources.

Cold Cuts

Some women opt to give up deli meats altogether during pregnancy, as they can harbor invisible, odorless bacteria like *Listeria*, which can cause miscarriage. If you just can't quit them, that's okay—just always cook them and eat 'em while they're piping hot.

Unpasteurized Milk

It (and its offspring, like unpasteurized yogurt or kefir) may contain bacteria such as *Campylobacter*, *E. coli*, *Listeria*, or *Salmonella*. Just say no to the cute, home-bottled stuff at the farmers' market, and buy pasteurized moo juice instead.

Unpasteurized Soft Cheeses

Check the label on that goat cheese, Brie, feta, Camembert, Roquefort, queso blanco, or queso fresco: If it says "un-pasteurized," it may contain *E. coli* or *Listeria*. The good news, though? Most cheese in the United States—yes, even most grocery-store brands of stinky Brie!—are pasteurized and good to go.

Unpasteurized Juice or Cider

Sensing a theme here? Juices that haven't undergone the bacteria-zapping process may contain *E. coli*, which could make you very sick. If your well-meaning cousin brought over a jug of fresh apple cider, bring it to a rolling boil on the stove and boil for at least one minute before drinking. (Insider tip: Add some cinnamon sticks to the mix while you're at it. Cinnamon has been shown to help the body manage its blood sugar levels more effectively—and it's delicious!)

Raw Cookie Dough or Cake Batter

Alas: The raw egg may contain *Salmonella*. That doesn't mean you need to give up fresh-baked cookies— just your desire to lick the spoon.

Shark, King Mackerel Swordfish, and Tilefish

They may contain high levels of mercury. Instead, reach for fish and shellfish that are lower in mercury, such as salmon, pollock, catfish, and shrimp.

Raw or Undercooked Seafood

Cook it at 145 degrees Fahrenheit (a meat thermometer is a great investment right now), and pass on sushi and oysters. Uncooked fish may contain parasites or bacteria.

Meat Salads

Ham salad, chicken salad, seafood salad, anything meaty that's kept in the fridge is a bad idea when you're browsing the deli counter, as they may contain *Listeria*. If you're eating meat, always make sure it's cooked and steaming before you dig in.

Raw or Undercooked Sprouts

Alfalfa sprouts, clover sprouts, mung bean sprouts, and radish sprouts are all banned from your salads and sandwiches for the time being, as they may contain *E. coli* or *Salmonella*. Thoroughly cooked sprouts get the A-OK, though.

Unpasteurized Eggs

Unless they're fully, firmly cooked. Like a runny egg yolk? Always use eggs that are marked as pasteurized. If you're eating out, it's best to stick to a fully, firmly cooked variety to avoid *Salmonella*.

Medium–Rare Anything

Much as you might like a little pinkness, undercooked meat may contain *E. coli*. Cook beef, veal, and lamb steaks to 145 degrees Fahrenheit; pork and all ground meats should hit 160 degrees Fahrenheit.

Undercooked Poultry

It may contain *Campylobacter* or *Salmonella*, so cook that chicken breast or turkey burger to 165 degrees Fahrenheit.

Smoked Seafood

Take a pass on lox at the bagel counter. Smoked, refrigerated seafood is iffy because you have no guarantee the meat got hot enough to kill off bacteria—and even if it did, bacteria could have lurked back in during the cooling process. Opt for a canned version, which is safe, or cook the fish to 165 degrees Fahrenheit before eating.

Sausage, Hot Dogs, or Cured Deli Meats

These types of meat contain nitrates; once inside our bodies, these chemicals are converted to nitrosamines, which have been found to increase your risk of developing cancer. Desperate for bacon? Go for a brand that isn't cured with chemical nitrites, like Applegate Naturals Uncured Sunday Bacon. If sausages and bologna are a regular part of your lunch menu, consider switching to well-cooked chicken burgers or steaming hot sliced turkey melts for the duration of your pregnancy.

Partially Hydrogenated Oils (trans fats)

The American Heart Association says the limit of what you should have is 2 grams a day, and most doctors prefer that you eat absolutely no trans fats. Why? Not only are they bad for your heart, but they're super bad for your pregnancy. According to one study, pregnant women who ate the most trans fat were seven times more likely to experience preeclampsia. And a diet high in trans-fats during pregnancy and breast-feeding could affect the growth of your baby's brain and eyes, because they block omega-3 fatty acids.

THE VICE SQUAD

In a world where everyone thinks they know best, you just need to know the truth.

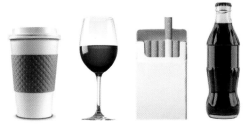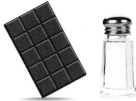

It's insane and wrong and sad, but all too true—once people know you're expecting, many of them will feel like they have the right to mandate your behavior, your diet, and your choices. Everyone has their own opinions—and own stories about what worked and what didn't during their pregnancies—but that doesn't mean you should listen to their chatter. It's still your body, after all!

I want you to be able to live your life and make food choices just like you always would—with confidence (no matter what that nosy checkout lady at the supermarket decides to warn you against this week!). That's why I talked to experts and dug through the research to separate fact from fiction.

COFFEE
Fine In Moderation

The American College of Obstetricians and Gynecologists has given the green light to having 200 mg or less of caffeine a day. So go ahead and have one or two small, 8 ounce cups of coffee—that's the equivalent of two short cups or one grande at Starbucks. If you want to be extra cautious, try decaf—you'll still get a tiny dose of caffeine, plus the placebo effect of sipping on some java.

ALCOHOL
Really Bad

About one in 13 moms-to-be drink—whether it's having an occasional celebratory glass of wine, a regular nightcap, or a more serious struggle with alcohol dependency. And despite what you might have heard, new research suggests that all of these scenarios can harm your baby. If you've had a drink or two since learning you were pregnant, don't panic, but you truly should think twice

before you have another. As many as 1 in 5 American children, many of whom seem happy and healthy, could have one of the fetal alcohol spectrum disorders (FASD), according to a large study in the journal *Pediatrics*—way above the old estimate of 1 percent of the U.S. population. These effects might be subtle, like ADHD or lower-than-average height or weight, but they can also include heart defects, changes in the shape of the face, poor muscle tone and problems with balance, problems with thinking and speech, and learning difficulties. No glass of vino is worth all that worry.

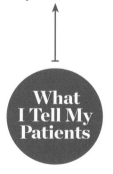

What I Tell My Patients

SMOKING
Really Bad

We all know that smoking dramatically increases your risk for lung, cervical, throat, and mouth cancers, plus heart disease, lung disease, stroke, and osteoporosis. So you know you have to quit. Now's the time: When a baby is exposed to cigarettes in the womb, it decreases the amount of oxygen in his blood, stunts his growth, and increases the chance that he'll be born too early and will develop asthma, ADHD, or other cognitive/behavioral problems or even suffer from Sudden Infant Death Syndrome

(SIDS). If you can't kick butt on your own, ask your health-care provider to help you find a smoking cessation program that will work for you.

SODA
Pretty Bad

Unless you reach for a decaffeinated soda, there's the caffeine issue again. But more importantly, sodas are a source of empty calories, and inject your system with sugar—which is not, you'll note, one of the key nutrients your developing body needs. In fact, one Norwegian study of more than 60,000 pregnant women showed that

Most OBs and their professional communities (ACOG, the CDC, the AAP) say avoid alcohol entirely, for a very simple reason: There is zero risk associated with abstaining from alcohol, but there are risks associated with drinking. So from a purely statistical and scientific standpoint, counseling total abstinence makes sense. But being realistic, for a special occasion or in the 3rd trimester, a sip or two isn't likely to do any damage.

those who drank one sugary soda a day were about 25 percent more likely to give birth prematurely than those who skipped the drink. And diet sodas aren't the answer—artificially sweetened sodas seem to increase the risk of preterm birth, too. A safer bet: seltzer with a few fruit slices or a splash of juice.

SUGAR
Pretty Bad

Too much sugar has been linked to everything from heart disease to diabetes to cancer to obesity. In 2011, Harvard scientists who had been following more than 120,000 people for between 12 and 20 years announced that sugar-sweetened beverages were among the foods most closely linked to long-term weight gain.

CHOCOLATE
Totally Safe

Eating well during pregnancy needn't mean giving up your favorite candy! A Yale study found that expectant moms who ate chocolate five or more times a week were 70 percent less likely to develop preeclampsia compared to those who ate it less than once a week. Dark chocolate, in particular, contains a substance thought to have cardiovascular benefits that help prevent preeclampsia—plus, it's a great source of iron, which you need more of right now to help carry oxygen to your growing baby.

ARTIFICIAL SWEETENERS
Pretty Bad

Some scientists suspect that nonnutritive sweeteners actually promote weight gain because of how we metabolize them. Consider artificial sweeteners like Splenda (sucralose), Equal (aspartame), and Truvia (stevia leaf extract) as no better than refined sugar: they're probably fine in moderation, but they're absolutely not a free pass to gluttony.

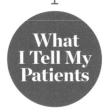

What I Tell My Patients

The World Health Organization recommends limiting one's intake of added sugars—that includes not just sugar but high fructose corn syrup, honey, agave syrup, maple syrup, and all the many chemistry-set-like ingredients such as sucrose, maltodextrin, and the like—to no more than 25 grams a day. And I agree. That means you're making ice cream, cookies, candy, and other sugary treats a rare indulgence; eliminating sugary beverages entirely; and checking the labels to make sure foods like pasta sauce, peanut butter, and salad dressings don't have added sugar (most do).

SALT
Pretty Bad

You already know that salt has long been considered a factor in high blood pressure. But recently, some researchers have come to suspect that high-sodium foods may also lead to unhealthy weight gain—and not just from the bloating that often accompanies salty meals. A 2015 study in the journal *Hypertension* found that the more salt a person eats, the more they are likely to weigh, regardless of calorie intake.

FRIED FOODS
Sometimes Bad

If it's not clearly fried in olive oil, you can bet it's fried in something bad. When you hanker for fried foods, cook them at home. In a 2016 study in the journal *Food Chemistry*, researchers from the University of Granada in Spain cooked potatoes, pumpkin, and eggplant using a variety of methods, including frying and boiling. The researchers found that when the vegetables were fried in olive oil, their levels of phenolic compounds—antioxidants that are shown to protect against cancer and slow the aging process—actually increased. That's right: Fried foods are good for you, as long as they're fried in the good stuff.

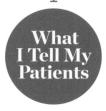

What I Tell My Patients

The average American woman eats 2,980 mg of sodium a day, and if that sounds like a lot, it is: You could eat a dozen of those little salt packets from McDonald's and still not approach that level. But most of the salt we eat comes not from the shaker, but from processed and restaurant foods.

THE **EAT THIS, NOT THAT!**
ESSENTIALS CHECKLIST

Proteins

You've heard of "Lean In." With meat, you'll want to "Think lean."

Chicken

Turkey

Pork Loin

Eggs

Tofu

Lean beef
(like lean ground beef, sirloin, or flank steak, grass-fed if possible)

Fish

The wilder, the better—but avoid fish high in mercury, like tilefish and shark.

Wild salmon
(also try "bone-in")

Cod

Halibut

Pollock

Wild mackerel

Sardines

Clams
(well-cooked)

Atlantic herring

Light canned tuna

Dairy

When buying milk and cheese, look for "pasteurized," not "un-pasteurized."

Milk
(1% pasteurized)

Yogurt
(low in sugar)

Cheese
(pasteurized)

Cottage cheese

Kefir

Dairy alternative:
almond milk
(unsweetened, ideally without carrageenan)

Fruits

The fruit of your labor will love these.

Apples

Bananas

Citrus fruits
(oranges, grapefruits, lemons, limes, tangerines)

Mango

Strawberries

Cantaloupe

Kiwi

Figs

Prunes

Vegetables

Dig into these high-nutrient picks.

Dark, leafy greens
(spinach, collard greens, kelp, Romaine lettuce, endive, swiss chard)

Sweet potatoes

Peas

Tomatoes

Brussels sprouts

Broccoli

Broccoli rabe

Avocado

Okra

Asparagus

Shiitake and **Portobello mushrooms**

Winter squash

Red and **green bell peppers**

Corn on the cob

Kimchi

Legumes

The darker the bean, the sweeter the nutrition.

Kidney beans

Navy beans

White beans

Lentils
(especially red)

Chickpeas

Pasta

Look for brands that are "enriched."

Whole wheat pasta—any shape or size

Grains

Go wild—or brown—for the best choice.

Wild rice

Brown rice

Quinoa

Cereals

Don't buy any with a cartoon animal on the box.

Oatmeal
(unsweetened)

Fortified cereal
(low in sugar)

Breads

Yes, you can eat carbs while pregnant! If they're whole grain.

Whole wheat bread

Corn tortilla

Seeds

These will increase your fiber optics— and go great in smoothies.

Sunflower seeds

Pumpkin seeds

Chia seeds

Flax seeds

Oils

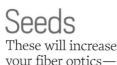

Go ahead, get "fat" while pregnant— as long as they're healthy fats.

Olive oil

Canola oil

Sesame seed oil

Grapeseed oil

Coconut oil

Avocado oil

Flaxseed oil

Nut oils

Cod liver oil

Fish oil

Nuts

A handful has healthy oils.

Peanuts

Walnuts

Almonds

Brazil nuts

Pistachios

Spices

Most spices are healthy, but hotter ones may cause indigestion.

Table salt
(as opposed to sea salt, which has no iodine, a hormone balancer)

Ground mustard and mustard seeds

Spreads

Go low or no-sodium, and sugar-free.

Nut butters

Sweets

For when the craving strikes...

Dark chocolate
(70% cacao or more)

Teas

All teas have benefits, but this one might help milk production.

Nettle Tea

Juice

Fruit juice is liquid sugar; if you want one, go with...

Tomato juice

Chapter

2

The First Trimester Diet

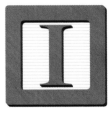**N THE FIRST TRIMESTER,** your baby is teeny-tiny inside you, a sprite-like hitchhiker who takes up hardly any room in your undercarriage. In fact, you likely won't even be showing yet—handy if you're trying to keep your news under wraps. And while you may not *feel* totally perfect (even just one day without nausea would be amazing, right?), these three months are a time to start laying the groundwork for a perfect diet—one that will not only form the basis of your pregnancy nutrition plan, but can see you through a lifetime of healthy eating.

That's because in the first 12 weeks, you don't need to ramp up your food intake at all; the healthiest first trimester diet is a healthy diet, period. (After the first 12 weeks, you'll need about 300 extra calories a day—but we'll get to that later). So think of this chapter as your ultimate healthy eating resource, for now *and* after baby makes her grand entrance.

So, what does a healthy diet look like, anyway?

Here's an easy outline to follow:

CALORIES

Aim for approximately 1,800 a day, enough to keep your weight stable for the first trimester (or to help you slowly lose weight after baby's arrival).

MEALS

Three meals a day, including—and yes, it is the most important of all—breakfast. A study at Tel Aviv University found that people who skip breakfast experience dramatic swings in blood-sugar levels after lunch and dinner—no matter how healthy those meals are. As a result, skipping breakfast will put you at greater risk for weight gain, diabetes, and general fatigue and crankiness.

SNACKS

Try to limit big snacks to the afternoon; studies show that people who snack in the P.M. gain less weight than those who snack before noon.

MEAL CHECKLIST

With every meal or snack, ask yourself:

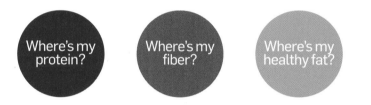

Where's my protein? Where's my fiber? Where's my healthy fat?

FOODS TO FOCUS ON

Lean Meats & Fish (protein, healthy fat)

Poultry, lean beef, and fish that are low in contaminants are your best choices for keeping your metabolism-boosting protein levels high.

Eat This! Wild salmon, tuna, halibut, sardines, lean beef, chicken, turkey, duck, roast pork

Not That! Processed meats and meats that are breaded, fried, or that use fillers (like chicken nuggets, hot dogs, and sausages); high-contaminant fish like tilapia, swordfish and shark.

Beans & Legumes (protein, fiber)

Lentils and beans carry the essential vitamins and minerals your body needs, plus fiber and protein to help keep you full.

↻ *Eat This!* Darker beans such as black and kidney beans have higher levels of vitamins and minerals, while Navy beans are packed with omega-3 fatty acids

↻ *Not That!* It's hard to screw up a bean. Look for low-sodium if choosing canned.

Nuts & Seeds (protein, fiber, healthy fats)

Rich in healthy fats, protein, and fiber, nuts and seeds are the most complete foods around. Eat more.

↻ *Eat This!* Walnuts, almonds, Brazil nuts, pistachios, and peanuts are among the most healthful, although all nuts have their virtues. Peanut, cashew, and almond butter are also great choices.

↻ *Not That!* Nut butters with added sugar; candied nuts

Vegetables & Fruits (fiber)

You need a wide variety throughout the day in order to keep your vitamin and mineral levels high. Mix up a variety of colors and flavors, and try to have at least one serving of fruit or vegetable at every meal.

↻ *Eat This!* Every whole fruit or vegetable you can get your hands on. As for juices, remember that they have had their natural fiber stripped out, and aren't nearly as healthy as the real thing; drink them in moderation.

↻ *Not That!* Fruit juice cocktails with added sugars; canned or dried fruit

Whole grains (fiber)

There's a whole-grain version of just about everything, from bread to pasta to crackers. Always look for the words "100 percent whole grain" so you know you're getting the healthy vitamins, minerals, and fiber that come with these complete grains.

⟳ *Eat This!* Brown rice, whole-wheat bread, whole-wheat pasta, oatmeal, quinoa, corn on the cob, corn tortillas

⟳ *Not That!* White rice, white bread, plain pasta, sugary cereals, sugar-added oatmeal, flour tortillas

Oils & Healthy Fats (fats, of course)

Healthy oils keep you full and help your body metabolize the vitamins and minerals found in the rest of your foods.

⟳ *Eat This!* Olives and olive oil; canola, sesame seed, and grape seed oil; coconut oil; avocados and avocado oil; nuts and nut oils

⟳ *Not That!* "Vegetable" oil, or any oil made from corn or soybeans. These oils—used often in fried fast foods and pre-made baked goods because they're cheap—have been linked to inflammation and unhealthy weight gain.

Dairy (protein)

Your best source of calcium and vitamin D, both crucial for healthy weight management and overall health, as well as baby's development. While the U.S. government continues to recommend cutting down on saturated fat, many health organizations now question that logic. In a 2013 *European Journal of Nutrition* research review, 11 of the 16 studies included found that participants who consumed more high-fat dairy products gained less unhealthy weight over time than their counterparts who didn't consume fat-laden dairy. Other studies have found that the more fat your dairy contains, the lower your risk of diabetes. The key thing to remember with dairy foods is to pick plain, unflavored, unsweetened products, and then add fruit and other natural flavors yourself.

🔄 *Eat This!* Plain regular and Greek yogurt, milk, pasturized cheese, kefir

🔄 *Not That!* Fat-free dairy, flavored dairy (e.g., "fruit on the bottom" yogurt), processed cheeses (like American cheese and Cheez Whiz)

———————————————————————

All that said, many women feel ravenous during their first trimester. To keep yourself from grabbing the closest thing to you (hello evil office vending machine!), start making it a habit to store a healthy snack in your bag before you head out the door: a handful of almonds; a pot of hummus and some veggies; or an apple and a squeeze pack of peanut butter. As your pregnancy progresses, you'll naturally start to eat smaller meals and snack more: You'll be hungry more often, but it'll become tricky to eat as much in one sitting since your growing uterus will make you feel full faster. A benefit: Smaller plates are less likely to give you reflux, a common preg side effect.

Throughout this book, we'll be keeping an eye on sodium for you, and trying to limit your intake to no more than 1,000 mg at any given meal. When you're eating out, especially in our country's most popular restaurants, where entrees commonly top 3,000 mg each (at P.F. Chang's, one order of Hot & Sour Soup delivers 7,980 mg!), that's not always possible. So we've highlighted some lower sodium items, even though they might go over the ideal limit. Look to keep your daily intake to not more than 2,300 mg.

Sample Daily Menu / First Trimester

Breakfast

1 cup vitamin D–fortified whole grain cereal
with quarter cup of blueberries, half a dozen almonds, and 8 ounces of almond milk.

339 calories
7 g fat (0 g saturated)
433 mg sodium
7 g fiber
23 g sugars

Lunch

Grilled Chicken Salad
with romaine lettuce, avocado, carrots, pumpkin seeds, balsamic vinaigrette—make sure the chicken is served steaming hot!

Yogurt smoothie with 1 banana, 1 tbsp peanut butter, ½ cup Greek yogurt, ¼ tbsp honey, ice, and water to blend

723 calories
37 g fat (6 g saturated)
556 mg sodium
9 g fiber
29 g sugar

Snack

2 ½ cups popcorn
air popped, salted, with ½ tbsp olive oil on top

137 calories
8 g fat (1 g saturated)
583 mg sodium
3 g fiber
0 g sugar

Dinner

Salmon, Rice, and Greens Bowl
Baked wild salmon, brown rice, and steamed spinach and kale

599 calories
13 g fat (2 g saturated)
118 mg sodium
5 g fiber
0 g sugar

GRAND TOTAL = 1,798 calories / 65 g fat (9 g saturated) / 1,690 mg sodium / 24 g fiber / 52 g sugar

How Much Weight Should a Mom-to-Be Gain?

The next nine months are critical not only for your baby's future health, but for yours as well. Staying in a healthy weight range is the best way to ensure that you'll have the energy and health to be the vibrant, involved mother you always dreamed of being. A large study published in *Public Health Nutrition* found that how many extra pounds you'll be carrying around 15 years from now— and all the negative health consequences that go along with them—hinges less on your pre-pregnancy figure and more on how many pounds you put on in these crucial nine months.

Women who are of healthy weight when they conceive but who go on to gain too much may confront another set of problems: gestational diabetes, high blood pressure, and even preeclampsia (a dangerous condition characterized by high blood pressure, fluid retention, and loss of protein through urine). And several large studies hint that gaining too much (or too little!) weight during pregnancy ups your offspring's risk of developing obesity during childhood.

Every baby, and every mom, is different, but the American College of Obstetricians and Gynecologists has some guidelines on how much weight pregnant women should gain. ACOG bases these guidelines on a woman's pre-pregnancy weight. (Note: These guidelines are for women carrying a singleton, not for women having twins or multiples.) To figure out where you stand, you'll need to calculate your Body Mass Index, or BMI.

The BMI is a formula that takes into consideration your height and your weight, and gives you a decent indication of whether you're overweight, obese, or in good shape. Type "BMI calculator" into a search engine, and you'll find

Heavy Matters

You might have wondered why women aim to put on 25 to 35 pounds (on average) when a newborn weighs a teeny fraction of that. The truth is, the extra poundage comes from a number of changes your body makes to bring your son or daughter into the world. All that extra blood you're packing to deliver oxygen to your baby, plus your breast growth, the amniotic fluid, and baby's placenta will weigh you down!

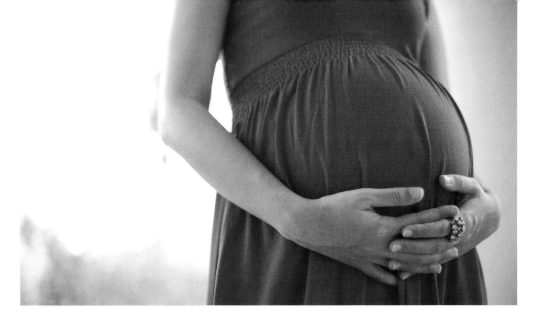

one easily. Once you've calculated your starting BMI, you can start tracking your pregnancy weight gain.

18.5 to 24.9: *Healthy Weight*
You should put on a total of 25 to 35 pounds—gaining just under a pound a week in the second and third trimesters.

25 to 29.9: *Overweight*
You should gain 15 to 25 pounds—gaining a little over half a pound per week in the second and third trimesters.

30 or above: *Obese*
Don't panic. Pregnancy may give you the perfect inspiration to bring your BMI back under control, and to begin eating in a way that sets you and your child up for a healthier, happier future. Many experts say you should gain 11 to 20 pounds total, adding just a half-pound per week in the second and third trimesters, but if you are in this range, it's crucial that you talk to your doctor about your

weight-gain goals during pregnancy. Now is not the time to try out a new fad diet to drop those pounds! Your baby needs nutrients and your doctor can help you come up with a smart plan.

Less than 18.5: *Underweight*

If you're more slender than your doctor would like you to be, you should look to gain between 28 and 40 pounds—gaining a full pound per week in the last two trimesters. That sounds like a tall order, but it just means chowing down a tiny bit more: Underweight women need an additional daily snack of about 200 calories (that's on *top* of the 300 calories a normal-weight woman adds in her second and third trimesters) through all nine months to put on the targeted 28 to 40 pounds. If that's you, try a handful of almonds and raisins midmorning or a bowl of cereal and milk before bed, whether you're hungry or not. But again, talk to your doctor and follow her advice—she knows best!

Your OB will monitor your weight at every visit. If she thinks you're gaining too little or too much—or if morning sickness keeps you from eating what you should—she may refer you to a nutritionist to keep you on track. In fact, the latest research suggests that the kind of food you're eating is a better indication of your overall pregnancy health than the number you see on the scale. Moms-to-be who upped their consumption of fruits and vegetables and reduced the level of saturated fat in their diets had better outcomes for their baby after birth (including shorter hospital stays, healthier birth weights, and reduced risk of respiratory complications)—*regardless* of how much weight they gained during those nine months, according to a study from the University of Adelaide. In other words, your top job is to give your developing child the healthiest food possible; let your doctor pay attention to the number on the scale.

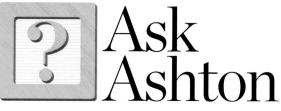

Ask Ashton

Why do I crave pickles and ice cream so often?
—Sara M., Calabasas, CA

Experts aren't sure why some women have selective cravings during pregnancy. There is a nutritional explanation for the pickles and ice cream, however. Pickles are incredibly salty. During pregnancy, plasma blood volume expands. The salt tends to draw water with it into the bloodstream, helping this process along. As for ice cream, it's high in dairy fat and sugar, which can activate your brain's reward centers. Enjoy it, but don't go overboard!

I'm vegan—and pregnant. My mother-in-law says I'm nuts to stick to my current diet. Is she right?
—Naomi B., Athens, GA

Big sigh of relief: It's safe to maintain an animal-free diet during pregnancy. If you're vegan, rely on cal-cium fortified soy or almond milk and dark leafy greens, since you won't nab calcium from the usual source, dairy. And watch your intake of iron and B vitamins, which omnivores often snag from meaty fare. (One study, published in the journal *Nutrition Reviews*, reported that 62 percent of vegetarian preggos are vitamin B12-deficient.)

I'm a coffee addict who's hoping to get pregnant soon. How much am I going to have to cut back?
—Shayna S., Southfield, MI

It depends on just how addicted you are. The American College of Obstetricians and Gynecologists notes that "moderate caffeine consumption [less than 200 milligrams per day] does not appear to be a major contributing factor in miscarriage or birth." That's one or two cups of coffee. But some studies suggest that caffeine is linked with low birth weight. A daily cup of joe is probably fine, but if you want to be extra cautious, try decaf—you'll still get a tiny dose of caffeine, plus the placebo effect of sipping on some java.

What can I eat in the morning that won't make me throw up?
—Bianca R., Lexington, KY

A good strategy is eating smaller, more frequent meals – including breakfast. Eggs can be very easy on the stomach and both mom and baby need some cholesterol for hormone production and cell development. You also get lots of protein and vitamin D in a small serving. Have just one or two eggs with a little whole-grain toast, and then follow up with some fruit a little later in the morning.

5 QUICK CRAVING CRUSHERS
Eat These with Ben or Jerry—Instead of Ben & Jerry's

4 Salty Snacks

2 Red Meat

1 Something Sweet

3 Tart Tastes

5 Comfort Food

ICE CREAM? Pulled pork? Pickle-and-peanut-butter sandwiches? As many as 9 out of 10 U.S. women experience food cravings during pregnancy, and many of them seem to come out of left field. These hankerings typically show up at the end of the first trimester, peak in intensity and frequency during the second trimester, decline through the third trimester, and then drop significantly after delivery.

The cravings you get when you're expecting are most likely to mimic the ones you've had in the past, especially when you were PMS-ing, according to a study published in the journal *Frontiers in Psychology*. Study participants who didn't have a history of cravings before pregnancy, on the other hand, were more likely to develop urges for salty, savory food, like pizza or fries, when they became pregnant.

Experts agree that impulses for certain foods stem from increased hormone production. While you're pregnant, your body will be churning out more than 30 different hormones, which in turn can lower your blood sugar (and lead to nausea), increase your metabolism (and boost hunger), and sharpen your sense of smell and taste (which can trigger morning sickness, food cravings, or food aversions).

Some pregnant women—scientists aren't sure how many—experience pica, a condition that makes them crave nonfood items such as dirt, paint chips, laundry starch, and other indigestible items. Doctors aren't sure why this happens (although they have found a link between pica and iron deficiency). What is certain is that giving in to these kinds of cravings *is* dangerous. If you find yourself hungry for something odd, talk to your doctor, who can discuss nutritional deficiencies and help you cope with the craving.

And here's a pregnancy myth that needs debunking: Craving a certain food during pregnancy—an iron-rich, juicy burger, say—probably does not mean your body is low in the particular nutrients it contains. True, many women are iron-depleted during pregnancy, but it's hard to show a cause-and-effect relationship between a craving and the lack of a specific nutrient. So be careful not to let cravings turn your first trimester into an

The Craving: Something Sweet
Food Fix: Banana-Chocolate Milkshake

YOU'LL NEED

1 **medium banana, frozen**

¾ **cup cold nonfat milk**

¾ **cups regular chocolate ice cream (not premium)**

½ **teaspoon chocolate syrup**

2-3 ice cubes

HOW TO MAKE IT

- In a blender, combine banana, ice and milk until smooth and frothy. Pour into a tall glass. Top with chocolate ice cream. Drizzle with chocolate syrup.

MAKES 1 SERVING

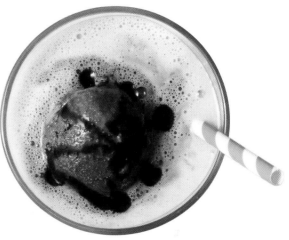

400 calories
20 g fat (12 saturated)
245 mg sodium
4g fiber
14 g protein

all-you-can-eat pickles and ice cream party: Research out of the UK notes that pregnant women who experienced food cravings took in more daily calories and gained more weight throughout their pregnancies than women who didn't. Instead, turn your cravings into opportunities to max out your top nutrients like calcium and folate. Here are five delicious and healthful recipes designed to satisfy the most common pregnancy cravings.

Craving: Red Meat
Food Fix: Big, Fat, Juicy Cheeseburger

YOU'LL NEED

½ medium onion, finely diced

1 teaspoon olive or grapeseed oil

1 cup finely diced portobello mushrooms

1 teaspoon balsamic vinegar

1 slice home-style white bread, crusts trimmed

1 teaspoon granulated garlic

¼ teaspoon paprika

1 pound 93 percent lean ground beef (7 percent fat)

Nonstick cooking spray

4 tablespoons loosely packed shredded sharp cheddar

1 cup loosely packed baby greens

4 whole-wheat hamburger buns

1 medium tomato, thinly sliced

1 small onion, thinly sliced

HOW TO MAKE IT

- In a small nonstick frying pan, sauté the diced onion in oil over medium heat until translucent, about 5 minutes. Add mushrooms and sauté for 1 minute, shaking pan. Turn heat up to high and add balsamic vinegar. Cook on high until vinegar is absorbed, about 30 seconds. Transfer to a large bowl and let cool.

- Meanwhile, place bread in a food processor and pulse until crumbs are formed. Transfer bread crumbs to bowl with mushroom mixture. Add garlic, paprika and beef. Using your hands, gently incorporate mushroom mixture into beef. (To avoid tough, dry burgers, do not over-handle meat.)

- Form into 4 patties, about 3 inches wide and 1 inch thick. Set a large frying pan on medium-high heat and lightly coat with nonstick spray. Place burgers in pan and cook for 5 minutes. Flip burgers and cook for 4 minutes more. Top each burger with a tablespoon of shredded cheddar. Cover frying pan and cook burgers an additional 2 minutes, until cheese has melted.

- Place about ¼ cup baby greens on each bun bottom, then top with tomato and onion. Place burger over onion and cover with bun top.

MAKES 4 SERVINGS

462 calories
17 g fat (6 saturated)
700 mg sodium
4 g fiber
50 g protein

Craving: Tart Tastes
Food Fix: Chicken Spinach Salad with Apple Dijon Vinaigrette

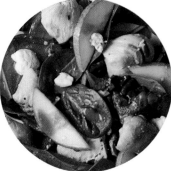

YOU'LL NEED

Dressing

- 4 tablespoons frozen apple-juice concentrate, thawed
- 2½ tablespoons balsamic vinegar
- 2 tablespoons Dijon mustard

Salad

- 1 teaspoon plus 1½ teaspoons olive oil, divided
- 1 teaspoon dried thyme
- 4 4-ounce boneless, skinless chicken breasts, cut into bite-size pieces
- Salt and pepper to taste
- 12 cups spinach leaves, torn
- 2 ripe pears, cored and thinly sliced
- ½ cup golden raisins
- 12 pecan halves, toasted and coarsely chopped
- 2 tablespoons pasteurized goat cheese, crumbled

432 calories
16 g fat (4 saturated)
276 mg sodium
7 g fiber
38 g protein

HOW TO MAKE IT

- To make the dressing: Whisk together apple-juice concentrate, vinegar, and mustard in a small bowl. Set aside.

- To make the salad: Warm 1 teaspoon oil in a large nonstick skillet over medium-high heat. Add thyme and chicken; sauté for 4 minutes. Reduce heat to low and stir in dressing. Slowly stir in remaining 1½ teaspoons oil and season with salt and pepper. Turn off heat and cover skillet for 1 minute.

- Divide spinach among four plates and top with pears. Spoon a portion of the hot chicken mixture over each salad; top with raisins, pecans, and cheese.

MAKES 4 SERVINGS

Craving: Salty Snacks
Food Fix: Chickpea "Chips"

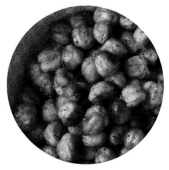

235 calories
7 g fat (1 g saturated)
512 mg sodium
10 g fiber
10 g protein

YOU'LL NEED

- **2 15-ounce cans chickpeas, drained**
- **1 tablespoon extra-virgin olive oil**
- **2 teaspoons Cajun spice mix**
- **1 teaspoon granulated garlic**
- **½ teaspoon dried oregano, crumbled**

HOW TO MAKE IT

- Preheat oven to 450° F. Place chickpeas and olive oil in a resealable plastic bag. Close bag and shake until chickpeas are coated with oil. (Not all the oil will be absorbed.) Place oiled chickpeas on a rimmed cookie sheet, then roast, occasionally turning with a spatula, until golden and crisp, about 45 minutes. Transfer roasted chickpeas to a serving bowl and toss with remaining ingredients. For best crunch, serve immediately.

MAKES 4 SERVINGS

Craving: Comfort Food
Food Fix: Two-Potato Mash

YOU'LL NEED

- 3 medium Yukon Gold potatoes, peeled and cut into ¾-inch cubes
- 2 medium sweet potatoes, peeled and cut into ¾-inch cubes
- 5 garlic cloves, peeled
- ½ cup low-fat buttermilk
- 1 tablespoon butter, cut into 4 pieces

HOW TO MAKE IT

- Fill a large stockpot with 3 inches of water, place a steamer basket in pot, and bring water to a boil. Reduce heat to low; place all the potatoes and garlic cloves in steamer basket and cover.

- Cook until tender, about 15 minutes. Run potatoes and garlic cloves through a food mill (or mash by hand) into a medium saucepan set over low heat.

- Add ¼ cup buttermilk and stir until incorporated. Add more buttermilk until desired consistency is reached. Toss in butter pieces, stir, and serve immediately.

MAKES 4 SERVINGS

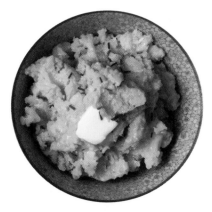

207 calories
3 g fat (2g saturated)
71 mg sodium
4 g fiber
5 g protein

EAT THIS, NOT THAT! Special Report

THE VEGAN PREGNANCY

If you live the cruelty-free life, now's the time when your family and friends might start laying on insane, unnecessary pressure: "But Honey, your baby needs protein! Have a burger!" They mean well, but um, come on. We are not living in the Stone Age, and there's no reason for you to give up your animal-free diet just because you're having a baby.

If you're vegan, rely on calcium-fortified nut milks and dark leafy greens, since you won't nab calcium from the usual dairy fare. And watch your intake of iron (key to producing red blood cells, which carry oxygen to baby) and B vitamins (including folic acid, crucial for preventing neural tube defects), which omnivores often snag from meat. One study, published in the journal *Nutrition Reviews*, reported that 62 percent of pregnant vegetarians are vitamin B12-deficient. Don't let that be you!

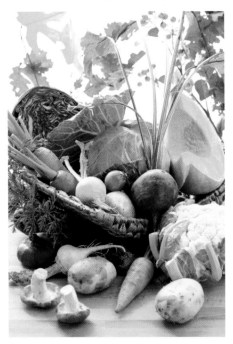

Vegetarians and vegans may also need to up consumption of omega-3 fatty acids (vital for Junior's cardiovascular health and brain and eye development) via fortified foods like juice or bread or algae supplements. Lastly, load up on legumes, nuts, and quinoa to get the extra 20 to 25 grams of daily protein you need—protein's amino acids are the building blocks of your little one's growth.

If you're not feeling healthy, though, don't hesitate to call your doctor. She may have specific dietary recommendations for you that can get you feeling better fast.

EATING FOR TWINS OR TRIPLETS

If you're a multiple mom-to-be, you've got a few things to consider. In addition to a larger car, a larger house, and a larger 529 savings plan, you're also going to need a larger dinner plate. Talk to your doctor about exactly how many calories you need, and how you can ensure you're getting the right mix of nutrients for your multiples.

Firm guidelines don't exist, but many experts say women pregnant with twins need an extra 500 calories per day in the second and third trimesters (versus the 300 bonus calories a woman pregnant with only one baby needs). A review article in the journal *Obstetrics & Gynecology* suggests you might need iron, folate, calcium, magnesium, and zinc supplementation beyond that contained in a typical prenatal vitamin, and possibly DHA or vitamin D supplements as well.

Carrying multiples also makes it more important to see consistent weight gain throughout your pregnancy, specifically before 28 weeks—this significantly decreases the risk of premature birth, increases birth weights, and reduces the risk of newborn death.

THE **EAT THIS, NOT THAT!**
MORNING SICKNESS SURV

Tossing your cookies into the trash can under your desk? Not cute. Or fun. Or helpful in keeping your news under wraps, for that matter. The relentless queasiness may be linked to increases in some hormones (such as estrogen), and to your heightened sense of smell—Mother Nature's way of making you hyper-vigilant about food safety. But whatever the cause, we know you just want it to go away already. Try these easy fixes and kick the barfy blues to the curb.

Eat Early

Stash some salty, 100 percent whole-grain crackers at your bedside and eat a few as soon as you wake up, even if you're not hungry. An empty stomach ups the risk of nausea.

Go for Balance

Aim for a diet high in protein (such as grilled chicken) and complex carbohydrates (such as whole grains and vegetables). If you start adding in rich, fatty foods, you may be more likely to suffer.

Grab a Lemon

Slice it, sniff it, squeeze it into your drinking water—the refreshing smell and taste can calm your stomach. Suck on lemon drops if you're feeling off while on the run.

Slurp Your Calories

If you're concerned about getting enough nutrients, try a broth-based soup or a smoothie, which will help both hydrate you and give you some calories when you don't feel like you can hold down solid food.

IVAL GUIDE

Meet Your New BFF, Ginger

It's no myth that ginger root can calm an upset tummy. Here's a soothing morning-sickness mocktail we love that puts the ingredient front and center:

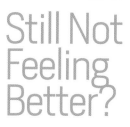

INGREDIENTS

4 to 6 raspberries (or 2 strawberries)

1 tablespoon lime juice

1 teaspoon grated ginger

¼ cup mango juice

¼ cup grapefruit juice

DIRECTIONS

- Muddle raspberries or strawberries at the bottom of a glass, and pour in lime juice. Add grated ginger, mango juice, grapefruit juice, and ice. Stir and enjoy!

85 calories
1 g fat (0g saturated)
7 g fiber
2 g protein

Still Not Feeling Better?

If your morning sickness is severe, you should talk to your doctor right away. She may recommend prescription medications like scopolamine, promethazine, prochlorperazine, or trimethobenzamide. (All have been shown to be safe for use during pregnancy.) If you can't hold liquids down for longer than 24 hours, you may be suffering from a more serious condition called hyperemesis gravidarum (yes, the same one that Kate Middleton famously suffered from), in which case you may have to be admitted to the hospital to be rehydrated. Just remember, no matter how dark things seem, you're not alone in this. And if you are worried about bothering your doctor, don't be! It's her job to make sure you are taken care of during this physically and emotionally charged time.

Chapter

3

The (Mildly Paranoid) Mom's Guide to Modern Chemistry

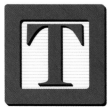

THE INCREDIBLE HULK. The Frankenstein Monster. The Real Housewives of Beverly Hills. Don't we have enough evidence already that when scientists fool around with biology, things can go really, really wrong?

Research shows that an estimated 739 chemicals can be found in our urine, blood, fat, brain, muscle, and bone. And more than 200 of those chemicals have been determined to have an effect on the human brain—yet most are not regulated, even to protect pregnant women and their unborn children. So, what's real? What's just hype?

We've taken the most worrisome substances, and sussed out whether each should be 100 percent **AVOIDED** or used on a limited basis with **CAUTION**. The fact is, some of these chemicals can't be completely avoided; they are in our environment and they are here to stay. But it might be possible to reduce your exposure, and in some cases you can even load your diet with nutrients that will mitigate any ill effects on you and your growing baby.

Make sure I'm BPA-free!

Bisphenol-A (BPA) › *Must Avoid*

WHAT IT IS:

This chemical was originally developed in the 1930s as an early estrogen replacement therapy. Today it's used to make polycarbonate plastics, mostly the hard clear shiny kind. It's commonly used to coat cans and bottle tops. Most alarming is that, until fairly recently, baby bottles were made with BPA—meaning that used plastic baby bottles are one gesture of kindness you should not accept.

WHY IT'S BAD:

In one study, the NIH found that significant levels of BPA in pregnancy to be associated with children who later displayed behaviors such as depression and withdrawal, anxiety, and Oppositional/Defiant Disorder. Another study found that prenatal BPA exposure negatively affected lung function in kids up to five years old.

HOW TO KICK IT:

Use alternatives—glass, for instance —for drinking, eating, heating, and storing food and beverages.

We used to think that if you just stayed away from plastic marked with a 3 or 7 on the bottom, you'd be safe. No more.

Be careful with cans.

Unless it says that it's BPA-free, it may not be. Brands that don't use BPA in their products: Amy's, Annie's Homegrown, Lucini Italia, Muir Glen, Earth's Best Organic, Eden Organic, Health Valley, Seneca, Sprouts Farmers Market, and Tyson.

Don't heat plastic.

The National Institute of Environmental Health Sciences advises against microwaving polycarbonate plastics or putting them in the dishwasher, because the plastic might break down over time and allow BPA to leach into food. BTW, that means if you put warm milk into a plastic bottle, it might leach as well.

Make sure you're getting enough folate.

A study by Duke University researchers found that folate is protective against fetal exposure to BPA, at least in animal studies.

Lead > *Must Avoid*

WHAT IT IS:

Lead is a naturally occurring element, but its presence in our daily lives is totally unnatural. It lingers in the environment after decades of use in paint and other home building products. And, although it's rare in our country, it can sometimes be found in candy, makeup, glazed pots, and serving dishes. Most lead use has been outlawed in the United States, but according to ACOG, about 1 percent of women of childbearing age (15–49) have blood levels that exceed the threshold of 5 micrograms/dL.

WHY IT'S BAD:

Exposure to lead during pregnancy and breastfeeding can result in life-long health issues, including damage to your baby's brain, kidneys, and nervous system. Lead passes from mother to unborn baby, so if your levels are high, so are your baby's. Too much lead in your body can put you at risk for miscarriage, cause your baby to be born too early or too small, and may cause your child to have behavior or learning problems later.

HOW TO KICK IT:

Stay away from any sanding or repairs if you have an older home (or aren't sure).

Lead dust is so tiny that you can't see it. You could be breathing it and not even know it. Also, if a family member works around construction, have them remove shoes and clothing before coming into the house.

Get your calcium.

Foods rich in calcium, iron, and vitamin C can protect you from lead. Calcium foods include milk, cheese, and yogurt; foods high in iron include beans, meat, peas, spinach, eggs, and fortified cereal; vitamin-C-rich foods include oranges, orange juice, grapefruit, strawberries, and tomatoes.

Ditch the fancy plateware.

Lead can sometimes be found in pottery and utensils from Latin America, India, and the Middle East—as well as in pewter, leaded glass, and crystal. It's important to pay attention not only to what you're eating and drinking, but to what you're eating and drinking from!

Mercury > *Must Avoid*

WHAT IT IS:

Another naturally occurring element that got into our food supply thanks to industrial carelessness and ignorance. While it's found in small concentrations in most seafood, it collects and builds up in the flesh of large, predatory sea creatures like shark, swordfish, king mackerel, tilefish, and some species of tuna.

WHY IT'S BAD:

Prenatal ingestion of mercury has been linked with offspring who have serious impaired neurological development; problems with learning, memory, and cognitive development; and ADHD.

HOW TO KICK IT:

Know the bad fish from the good fish.

It's plain and simple—don't eat shark, swordfish, king mackerel, tilefish, or white albacore tuna.

Eat all the good fish you want!

Studies consistently show that women who eat more than two servings of fish per week have children with higher IQ and fine motor skills, most notably because of the omega-3 fatty acids in many fish that can promote your baby's brain development. So there is zero reason to avoid seafood.

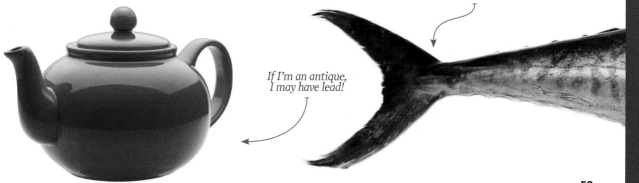

Throw me back in the water!

If I'm an antique, I may have lead!

Nitrates & Nitrites > *Must Avoid*

WHAT THEY ARE:

Chemical preservatives used to cure meats like hot dogs, bacon, bratwurst, and deli meat. Smaller amounts of nitrites and nitrates also get ingested through our drinking water, thanks to nitrogen-based fertilizers and livestock waste.

WHY IT'S BAD:

The World Health Organization has found that eating nitrite-containing meats increases your risk of cancer, and other organizations have found that consuming these meats while pregnant may be associated with increased incidence of brain tumors in children.

HOW TO KICK THEM:

Stay away from nitrite-rich bacon, hot dogs, and other cured meats

...in general, but especially while you're pregnant; any processed food deserves a glance at the label before you buy it.

Use a water filter.

(and change it regularly!) to remove nitrates and nitrites from your water. Look for a reverse osmosis system, which will filter out these and other chemicals such as arsenic, hexavalent chromium, and pharmaceuticals.

Check my package to ensure I'm nitrate-free!

Pesticides › *Caution*

WHAT THEY ARE:

A wide variety of natural and synthetic compounds that are used to combat bugs, fungus, and weeds.

WHY THEY'RE BAD:

DDT, the most harmful of pesticides, has been banned in the U.S. since 1972, but it is still widely used outside our country, both in agriculture and to control mosquitoes. DDT and its related compounds stick around in the environment for a long time: Recent UC Berkeley studies published in the journal Current Opinion in Pediatrics found that in utero exposure to DDT is associated with significantly diminished infant and child neuro-development.

HOW TO KICK THEM:

Choose organic when you can.
According to the EPA, modern synthetic pesticides are safer for human consumption, but genetically modified plants are designed to absorb more of these chemicals.

Filter your water.
Even banned pesticides can linger in groundwater for decades.

Buy American.
Choose produce from inside the U.S., which has higher environmental standards for pesticide use. In winter, look for frozen organic fruits, rather than imported versions from other countries.

Select a wide variety of fruits and vegetables.
so you won't be exposed to a concentration of any one pesticide.

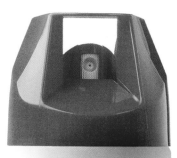

I might have been sprayed on your fruit!

Phthalates › *Must Avoid*

WHAT THEY ARE:

Phthalates are synthetic chemicals used in everyday items like soap, fragrance, and plastic toys (think rubber duckies—they make plastic pliable), and as ingredients in pesticides and food additives.

WHY THEY'RE BAD:

Phthalates are, without question, dangerous for pregnant women and their developing babies. *JAMA Pediatrics* states in a study published in 2014 that women exposed to phthalates during pregnancy have significantly increased odds of delivering preterm. In boys, phthalates damage the male reproductive system, decreasing testosterone levels and sperm count and quality. And in 2014 the journal *PLOS ONE* reported on a study that found high levels of phthalates in pregnant women correlated with deficits in their children's intellectual development later on.

HOW TO KICK THEM:

Choose whole, fresh foods that have been minimally processed, when you can.
Organic farming and practices might limit the amount of the substance that gets into food during production as well.

Do not heat plastic.
A "microwave safe" dish is not good enough, unless it's glass. Err on the safe side and just limit your exposure. Don't reheat leftovers in takeout containers and avoid microwaveable dinners that come in plastic packaging.

Remember to read labels
...especially those on your beauty and skin care products; and when you have the option, always opt for products that are labeled phthalate-free.

Buy products labeled "phthalate-free"!

Non-Stick Chemicals (PFOA)
> *Caution*

WHAT IT IS:

PFOA, an acronym for perfluorooctanoic acid, is a synthetic (man-made) chemical used extensively for more than half a century in things including carpets, textiles, and personal care products. You probably know them best for their use in non-stick cookware coatings such as Teflon.

WHY IT'S BAD:

PFOA appears to remain in the human body for a long time. A cohort study conducted with 665 Danish pregnant women and published in a 2012 Environmental Health Perspectives report found that PFOA exposure during pregnancy was associated with a higher risk of obesity for their children at 20 years of age. In animal studies, the EPA found that exposure to PFOAs caused problems such as preterm birth and low birth weight.

HOW TO KICK IT:

Toss the Teflon.

Although the EPA is maintaining that routine consumer use of non-stick cookware does not pose a problem, why risk it? Just use a cast iron skillet and some olive oil instead; you'll get the nutritional benefit of the sunny olive oil, and cooking in an iron skillet also boosts your iron consumption. At the very least, never use a metal utensil in a pan with a nonstick coating; scratching the coating allows the chemicals to seep into your food.

Goodbye for now!

Chapter

4

The Second Trimester Diet

VEN THOUGH, FROM THE OUTSIDE, it might seem like not much happens during the first trimester—you know better. Whether you've been battling nausea, headaches, mood swings, or any number of other unpleasant symptoms, getting through the first 12 weeks of pregnancy can be a bit of a bear. You. Deserve. A. Medal.

Now that you've gotten past many of those initial hurdles, you can bask in what many women call the "honeymoon phase" of their pregnancy. The morning sickness and fatigue that may have plagued your first trimester usually lifts during the second trimester, and you start to feel energetic and sexy (yes, sexy!) again. You're hopefully entering calmer waters, and can sail into the next phase of mamahood.

You also are probably starting to look more pregnant, too. While you might have gained just a few pounds during the first trimester, you'll find that the clothes you were still able to squeeze into aren't exactly fitting the same (if at all!) now. Celebrate your new figure with a few key pieces of maternity wear. You deserve to look and feel fabulous!

And this trimester is crucial to healthy weight gain: According to a study in the *American Journal of Clinical Nutrition*, underweight women who gained too little in the second trimester had a 72 percent likelihood of not gaining enough weight by their pregnancy's end, and heavy women who put on excess weight in this period had a 90 percent chance of gaining too much by their delivery date. I'll tell you a little more about why this is so important later in this chapter.

Your baby also is getting bigger. At the beginning of the 14th week, the fetus

Sample Daily Menu / Second Trimester

Breakfast

Peanut Butter & Raspberry Oatmeal with ½ cup rolled oats with 2 tbsp peanut butter and ½ cup raspberries

Banana chia pudding with 3 cups unsweetened almond milk and ½ cup chia seeds, mixed and refrigerated overnight. Top with ½ small banana, mashed and ½ tsp cinnamon. Makes 4 servings

613 calories
22 g fat (4 g saturated)
157 g sodium
24 g fiber
18 g sugar

Snack 1

3 tbsp peanuts, unsalted

240 calories
21 g fat (4.5 g saturated)
0 mg sodium
4.5 g fiber
1.5 g sugar

Lunch

Turkey avocado sandwich with 3 oz fresh roasted turkey breast, 1 cup arugula, ½ cup avocado, 2 tsp spicy mustard, and 2 slices sprouted grain bread

553 calories
19 g fat (4 g saturated)
377 mg sodium
11.4 g fiber
1 g sugar

Snack 2

Pumpkin pie smoothie with 1 cup skim milk, ½ cup unsweetened pumpkin puree, ½ cup nonfat frozen vanilla yogurt, 1 tbsp molasses, ½ oz nonfat powdered milk, and ½ tsp pumpkin pie spice, blended with ice

294 calories
0.5 g fat (0 g saturated)
247 mg sodium
4 fiber
41 sugar

Dinner

Chicken kebabs with quinoa and garbanzo beans Cut a chicken breast into 1-inch cubes and marinate in teriyaki sauce for 30 minutes. Put on skewer with chunks of zucchini, bell pepper, and onion. Grill until chicken is cooked through, about 6-7 minutes. Serve over cooked quinoa and garbanzo beans

2 skewers:
461 calories,
6 g fat (4 g saturated)
462 mg sodium
12.6 g fiber
8.6 g sugar

GRAND TOTAL = 2,161 calories / 68.5 g fat (16.5 g saturated) / 1,243 mg sodium / 56.5 g fiber / 70.1 g sugar

is about 4 to 4½ inches long and weighs about 2.5 ounces, the size of a medium apple; by week 28 she's growing fast, weighing in at more than 2½ pounds; she'll be at least 15 inches long and is almost as big as an eggplant. Her brain will increase in weight 400 percent to 500 percent between now and delivery. And she's starting to store calcium, iron, and phosphorus.

To support your baby's growth, you need between 300 and 400 more calories each day, for a total of roughly 2,200—but that number may be different for you, depending on your doctor's recommendations. To do it right, simply follow the guidelines we gave you in The First Trimester Diet, and add healthful snacks to make up the difference. The ideal way to add these additional calories is by focusing on fresh, whole foods that are low in sugar, high in protein and fiber, with moderate amounts of healthy fats.

SWEAT THIS, NOT THAT

While there's no need to sign up for a private trainer, staying active (or getting active if you've been a little inactive in recent years—no judgment!) is super important during pregnancy. Not only is it a great way to avoid packing on too many pounds—which of course can lead to pregnancy complications and have negative health effects on your little one down the road—exercise also helps increase the amount of oxygen you can deliver to your baby in the womb and can boost your mood. Oh, and one more thing? A jog around the block or dip in your local pool won't cost you a cent. Definitely talk to your doctor before starting any new workout regime, but barring any contraindications, experts say that pregnant women should work out moderately for at least 30 minutes on most days.

If you're looking for inspiration, walking, jogging, swimming, yoga, and weight lifting are great places to start.

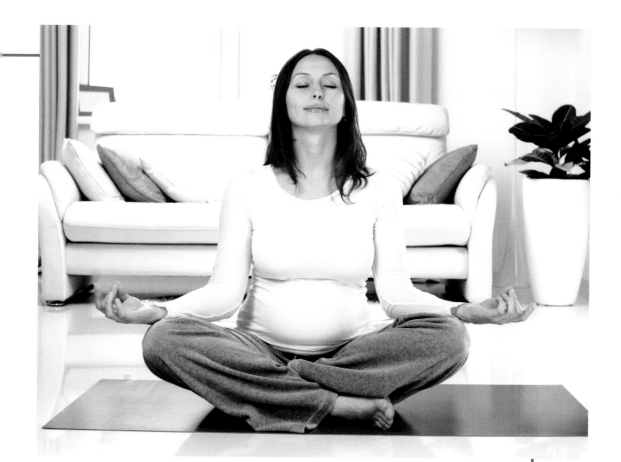

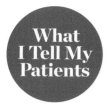

What I Tell My Patients

You can do almost anything you did before you got pregnant—with certain exceptions like scuba diving, hiking above 6,000 feet, and anything with a high risk of falling at a fast speed, such as downhill skiing and horseback riding. A good rule of thumb for cardio, weights, and other exercise: Don't add intensity or duration while you're expecting, and if you can't speak normally while you're exercising, you're pushing too hard. Stay hydrated and stop if you don't feel good. Simple!

The Fish-Hater's Guide to Omega-3s

Whether you're a vegetarian or simply just not into seafood, there are still plenty of ways to get the vital omega-3 fatty acids you need each day.

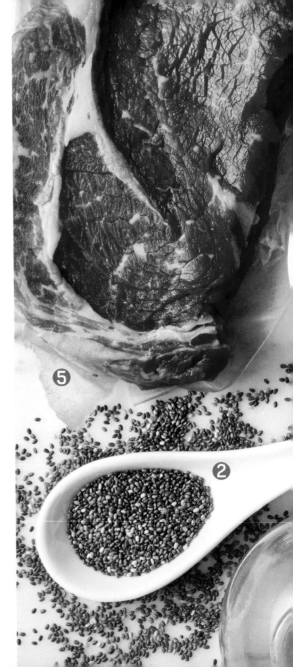

❶ WALNUTS
1 ounce (about ¼ cup) has 2.5 grams of ALA

Walnuts pack the most omega-3 punch of any nut or seed, and they're also high in disease-fighting antioxidants. This combination, according to a recent study, is highly protective against heart disease. Walnuts help reduce blood pressure and decrease inflammation in the blood vessels during times of stress.

❷ CHIA SEEDS
1 tbsp has 2.5 grams of ALA

Chia Pods and chia puddings are popping up in grocery stores and cafes for good reason—these seeds pack a major punch of nutrition! Try adding them to smoothies, stir fry, and more to give your meals an omega-3 boost. Even just a tiny shake each morning on your cereal ensures you're hitting your daily quota.

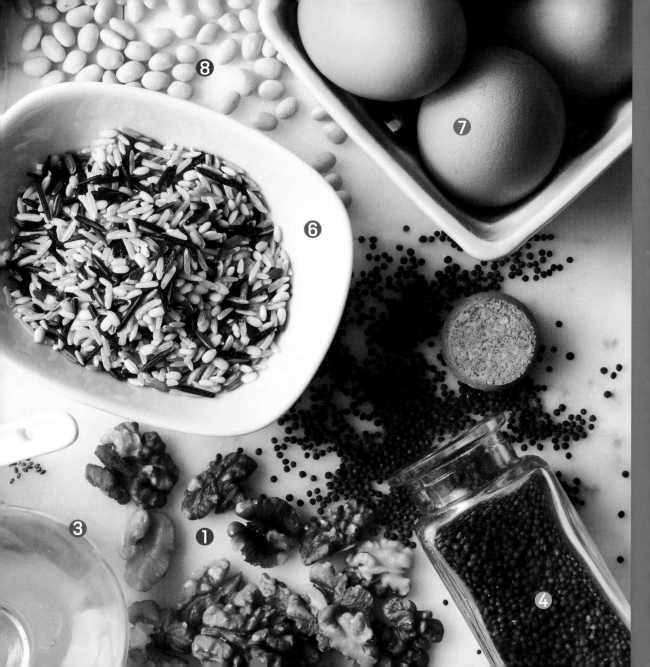

❸ FLAXSEED OIL
1 tbsp has 7.3 grams of ALA

While whole flaxseeds are high in ALA, their hard exteriors often resist digestion, meaning you don't always get the nutritional bang for your buck. Go for the ground version (also known as flax meal), which has about 2.3 grams of ALA per tbsp, or get nearly a week's worth of the good stuff by drizzling a little of the nutty-tasting oil onto your salad.

❹ MUSTARD SEEDS
1 tbsp has 0.2 grams of ALA

These little guys are loaded with omega-3s. Choose whole-seed mustard when you can, or use the seeds themselves in your cooking: You can sprinkle them into stir-fry, or toast them lightly and add them to pork dishes, yogurt curry dishes, and even salads.

❺ GRASS-FED MEAT
One 6-ounce steak has 0.16 grams of omega-3s

While red meat should definitely not be an everyday food, choosing grass-fed when you do indulge makes a big difference. Because they wander around in fields eating things like flax and purslane (about which you'll read, below), grass-fed cows yield meat that contains about 4 times more omega-3s than grain-fed animals.

❻ WILD RICE
½ cup has 0.3 g ALA

While not a common food in most of the U.S., this sour, slightly salty green is often used in Greek and Turkish cooking. A weed to most, it was a regular part of Gandhi's diet, and a mere half cup has more than 1,000 IUs of vitamin A—look for it at the Farmer's Market during spring and summer.

❼ OMEGA-3 EGGS
One Organic Valley Omega-3 Egg has 0.3 g ALA

Eggs turn up on many of our "best lists" because they are chock full of protein, vitamins, antioxidants, and a fat-fighting nutrient called choline. Omega-3 enriched eggs are laid by hens that are fed flaxseeds, chia seeds, and fish oil, automatically improving their nutritional content.

❽ NAVY BEANS
1 cup has 1.19 grams of ALA

Not only are beans a great source of belly-fat-fighting fiber, a single cup gives you an entire day's worth of omega-3s. Navy beans are packed with satiating protein and brimming with vitamins and minerals.

What's the Deal with Gestational Diabetes?

Even if you are healthy, eating nutrient- and fiber-dense foods and exercising, you still may be at risk for gestational diabetes mellitus (GDM). GDM is a state of relative glucose intolerance during pregnancy, meaning that your body may have trouble using the insulin it produces. When that happens, glucose gets essentially trapped in your bloodstream and isn't converted into energy—leading to both high blood pressure and feelings of sudden wooziness or fatigue.

High blood-sugar levels during pregnancy can lead to an oversized baby (or a severely undersized baby), as well as a baby with too much extra insulin in his system, which increases the risks of childhood obesity and Type II diabetes later in life.

Gestational diabetes often has no obvious symptoms, which is why it's important for your doctor to monitor your blood and to know your family history. Many OBs will perform an early screen for GDM in the first trimester for women who are obese, or who have a history of GDM in past pregnancies.

Otherwise, most pregnant women will be given a glucose tolerance test at around week 24. The test is simple: You'll be asked to drink a 50-gram glucose mixture, and your blood glucose will be measured one hour later. Should your blood glucose suggest you may have gestational diabetes, a three-hour glucose tolerance test will be performed.

If your doctor does find that you have the condition, it can be managed pretty easily, and it will likely subside after delivery (though you should also make certain you are re-checked approximately 6 to 8 weeks postpartum). Your doctor will most likely prescribe a specific meal plan and perhaps an exercise routine to help level things out.

SMART SNACKS
Delicious ways to get 350 extra calories a day

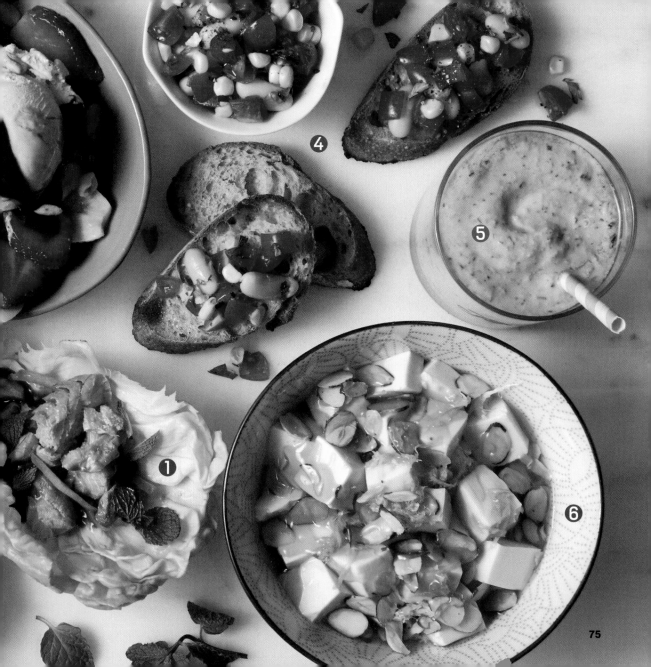

IF YOU'RE CARRYING ONE BABY, you'll need about 350 extra calories each day during the second trimester (if you're having twins, experts suggest 500 more daily). Take pleasure in those extra bites. You can choose simple snacks like hummus, pita and carrots or sugar snap peas; a peanut butter and jelly sandwich on whole grain bread; a handful of nuts; or an energy bar. Here are eight 350-calorie snacks that are easy to make, packed with pregnancy nutrients, and delicious, too.

❶ SALMON-HOISIN LETTUCE ROLLS

- 2 leaves of Bibb lettuce
- 1 tbsp hoisin sauce
- 6 oz drained canned salmon
- 1 small carrot
- Chopped mint

- Lay out lettuce leaves and spread each one with hoisin sauce.
- Scatter a 3-ounce portion of drained canned salmon over each leaf.
- Shred carrot, sprinkle over salmon, and top each portion with mint leaves.
- Roll up each lettuce leaf.

❷ WARM EGG AND SPINACH SANDWICH

- ¼ cup low-fat cottage cheese
- 1 Whole wheat English muffin
- ½ cup baby spinach
- 1 thick tomato slice
- 1 egg, scrambled
- ½ oz pesto

- Spread cottage cheese over each side of a toasted muffin.
- Top 1 muffin slice with baby spinach leaves and tomato slice.
- Top the other with a scrambled egg, pesto, and salt and pepper to taste.

❸ GRAB-AND-GO ENERGY MIX

- 2 cups All-Bran Extra Fiber cereal
- 2 cups fortified puffed wheat cereal
- 1 cup mini whole-wheat pretzels
- ⅓ cup dried cherries
- ⅓ cup dried currant
- ¼ cup toasted chopped walnuts
- ¼ cup raw pumpkin seeds
- 2 ounces cocoa nibs

- Combine all ingredients.
- Evenly divide mixture among 6 zip-top plastic bags.
- Makes 6 ½-cup servings.

❹ SUMMER VEGGIE CROSTINI

- **1 chopped ripe medium tomato with**
- **¼ cup cooked cannellini beans,**
- **2 tablespoons fresh, raw corn,**
- **2 tablespoons chopped fresh basil leaves,**
- **¾ teaspoon extra virgin olive oil, and**
- **½ teaspoon balsamic vinegar**
- **1 Whole wheat baguette**

- Combine the first six ingredients. Season with salt and pepper to taste and heap onto 2 ¼-inch thick slices of toasted whole-wheat baguette.

❺ ORANGE-BLUEBERRY LASSI

- **1 cup blueberries**
- **1 cup calcium-fortified orange juice**
- **6 ounces low-fat vanilla yogurt**
- **¼ teaspoon ground cardamom (or ginger)**
- **3 ice cubes**

- Whip up ingredients in blender.
- Serve in tall glass.

❻ MAPLE-GINGER TOFU "CRÈME CARAMEL"

- **8 oz block of silken tofu**
- **3 tbsp pure maple syrup**
- **¼ teaspoon freshly grated ginger**
- **2 tbsp sliced almonds**

- Place tofu in a small serving bowl.
- Pour maple syrup (heated, if desired) over tofu and top with ginger and almonds.

❼ PUMPKIN PIE SMOOTHIE

- **1 cup skim milk**
- **½ cup unsweetened pumpkin purée**
- **½ cup nonfat frozen vanilla yogurt**
- **1 tablespoon molasses**
- **½ ounce nonfat powdered milk**
- **½ teaspoon pumpkin pie spice**

- Whip up ingredients in blender.
- Serve in tall glass.

❽ LITE BANANA SPLIT

- **1 small banana**
- **½ cup sliced fresh strawberries**
- **2 tablespoons fat-free chocolate syrup**
- **½ scoop nonfat strawberry frozen yogurt**
- **½ ounce chopped roasted peanuts**

- Cut peeled banana lengthwise in half.
- Scoop frozen yogurt over the center of both halves and top with the rest.

6 Ways to Add 350 Healthy Calories to Your Day

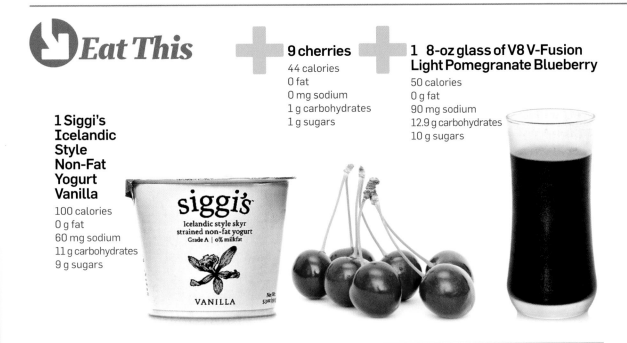

Eat This

+

9 cherries
44 calories
0 fat
0 mg sodium
1 g carbohydrates
1 g sugars

+

1 8-oz glass of V8 V-Fusion Light Pomegranate Blueberry
50 calories
0 g fat
90 mg sodium
12.9 g carbohydrates
10 g sugars

1 Siggi's Icelandic Style Non-Fat Yogurt Vanilla
100 calories
0 g fat
60 mg sodium
11 g carbohydrates
9 g sugars

This snack is packed with calcium from the yogurt, folate from the salad and plenty of vitamins and nutrients from the fruit; all of the sugars are natural fruit sugars.

In our 24/7, 7-Eleven culture, extra calories are never far from our hungry tummies. There are a million ways you could add 350 calories into your day, but the vast majority of them are pretty unhealthy. Here's a quick look at how much nutrient-rich food you can pack in for that calorie count—and how little junk food it takes to hit that number.

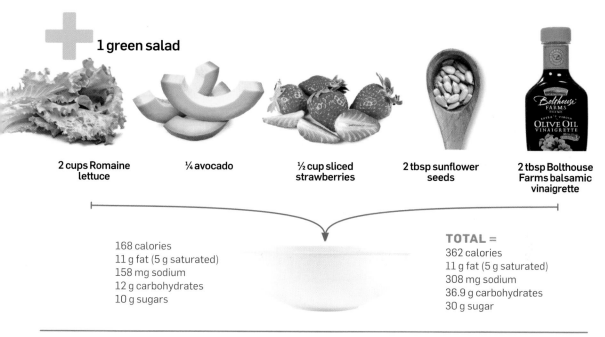

1 green salad

2 cups Romaine lettuce

¼ avocado

½ cup sliced strawberries

2 tbsp sunflower seeds

2 tbsp Bolthouse Farms balsamic vinaigrette

168 calories
11 g fat (5 g saturated)
158 mg sodium
12 g carbohydrates
10 g sugars

TOTAL =
362 calories
11 g fat (5 g saturated)
308 mg sodium
36.9 g carbohydrates
30 g sugar

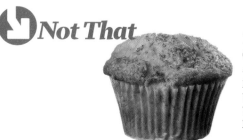

Not That

1 large corn muffin

424 calories
12 g fat (2 g saturated)
724 mg sodium
70 g carbohydrates
10 g sugars

This muffin may technically have fewer grams of sugar than the larger snack above, but all those carbs will be converted into sugars as well, leading to a massive crash later on.

Eat This

2 Kashi Blueberry Waffles

150 calories
5 g fat (0 saturated)
300 mg sodium
33g carbohydrates
4g sugars

Diced cantaloupe (½ cup)

30 calories
0g fat
28mg sodium
16g carbohydrates
14g sugars

1 Diana's Bananas Banana Babies Dark Chocolate

130 calories
6g fat (4g saturated)
15mg sodium
18g carbohydrates
14g sugars

1 8 oz glass of Langers Lite Cranberry Juice Cocktail

80 calories
0g fat
15 mg sodium
19 g carbohydrates
14 g sugars

TOTAL =
390 calories
11 g fat (4 g saturated)
358 mg sodium
86 g carbohydrates
46 g sugars

Don't get too hung up on the sugar count; most of it comes from nutrient-dense fruit sources—which are also full of amazing vitamins and nutrients you and your baby need.

Not That

½ cup Ben & Jerry's Peanut Butter Cup Ice Cream

370 calories
26 g fat (14 g saturated)
140 mg sodium
29 g carbohydrates
25 g sugars

Truth bomb? Although half a cup is the correct serving size for ice cream, most people serve themselves at least double that at home—so you might be getting even more junk than you think.

Eat This

Lifeway Lowfat Kefir Strawberry

140 calories
2 g fat (1.5 g saturated)
125 mg sodium
20 g carbohydrates
20 g sugars

2 kiwi fruit

92 calories
2 g fat (0 saturated)
8 mg sodium
44 g carbohydrates
26 g sugars

2 slices of Kashi Stone-Fired Thin Crust Pizza Mushroom Trio & Spinach

100 calories
7g fat (3g saturated)
495 mg sodium
21 g carbohydrates
2 g sugars

TOTAL =
332 calories
11 g fat (4.5g saturated)
628 mg sodium
85 g carbohydrates
48 g sugars

Organic and GMO-free, Lifeway Kefir is a drinkable yogurt that delivers 12 probiotic cultures; sipping the beverage can reduce bloating and gas brought on by lactose consumption by 70 percent, according to Ohio State University researchers. And don't overlook kiwis, which have 20 percent more vitamin C than oranges.

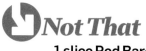

Not That

1 slice Red Baron Thin & Crispy Pepperoni Pizza

400 calories
18 g fat (8 g saturated)
1,010 mg sodium
42 g total carb
10 g sugars

The sodium levels in this will leave you feeling more bloated than a hot air balloon, plus—we all know processed meats like pepperoni increase your risk of developing cancer. Not exactly what you want to be feeding a developing baby!

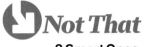

Eat This

Dannon Light & Fit Cherry Yogurt
80 calories
0 g fat
45 mg sodium
9 g carbohydrates
8 g sugars

½ banana
45 calories
0 g fat
1 mg sodium
23 g carbohydrates
12 g sugars

Applegate Farms Naturals Roasted Turkey Breast
on 1 Arnold Sandwich Thins Flax & Fiber, served hot
150 calories
1 g fat (0 g saturated)
530 mg sodium
21 g carbohydrates
0 g sugars

Lipton Brisk Lemon Ice Tea
80 calories
0 g fat
65 mg sodium
22 g carbohydrates
22 g sugars

TOTAL =
350 calories
1 g fat (0 g saturated)
641 mg sodium
75 g carbs
42 g sugars

Spreading these smaller snacks out throughout the day can help keep you at a steady energy level, even on the busiest, most hectic days.

Not That

2 Smart Ones Smart Anytime Mini Cheeseburgers
380 calories
9 g fat (4 g saturated)
360 mg sodium
20 g carbohydrates
4 g sugars

Foods with the word "smart" on the label are usually talking about reduced calories, but your job isn't primarily about managing calories—it's about packing in nutrition. Extra calcium and fruit, plus breads that are dense with fiber and nutrition, help the cause.

Eat This

1 Sargento Reduced Fat Sharp Cheddar Stick

60 calories
4.5 g fat (3 g saturated)
135 mg sodium
1 g carbohydrates
1 g sugars

10 strawberries

40 calories
0 g fat
0 mg sodium
10 g carbohydrates
10 g sugars

16 Tostitos Oven Baked Scoops
with 2 tbsp Newman's Own Mild Salsa

130 calories
3g fat (0.5 saturated)
191 mg sodium
24 carbohydrates
1 g sugars

Breyer's Black Raspberry Chocolate
(½ cup)

140 calories
4 g fat (3 g saturated)
35 mg sodium
25 g carbohydrates
16 g sugars

TOTAL =
370 calories
11.5 g fat (6.5 saturated)
361 mg sodium
60 g carbs
28 g sugars

Crunchy, creamy, cheesy—you can have it all if you pick wisely, and rack up plenty of extra calcium and micronutrients as well. Or you can blow it all on one nutrition-free snack.

Not That

15 Lay's Garden Tomato & Basil Potato Chips
with 3 tbsp Marzetti Dill Veggie Dip

330 calories
28 g fat (6g saturated)
425 mg sodium
25 g carbohydrates
10 g sugars

Both the Lay's and the Marzetti seem to indicate they're full of vegetables, but mostly you're just getting plain old fatty potato chips and sour cream.

Eat This

Gnu Foods Flavor & Fiber Banana Walnut Bar

140 calories
4 g fat (0 saturated)
40 mg sodium
30 g carbohydrates
8 g sugars

+

Spinach salad

1 cup spinach with 4 sliced strawberries, 1 oz crumbled feta cheese (make sure it's pasteurized) and Bolthouse Farms Classic Balsamic Olive Oil Vinaigrette

140 calories
6 g fat (4 g saturated)
490 mg sodium
12 g carbohydrates
9 g sugars

+

8 oz serving of AriZona Green Tea with Ginseng and Honey

70 calories
0 g fat
20 mg sodium
18 g carbohydrates
17 g sugars

TOTAL =
350 calories
10 g fat (4 g saturated)
550 mg sodium
60 g carbohydrates
34 g sugars

All the fiber in these snacks will help you avoid uncomfortable tummy troubles and keep you feeling full all day long.

Not That

Jamba Juice Strawberry Surf Rider
(16 oz)

320 calories
1 g fat (0 g saturated)
10 mg sodium
78 g carbohydrates
70 g sugars

This smoothie is made with sherbet—which isn't much healthier for you than ice cream. Make sure you know what's in the blender before you sip that drink!

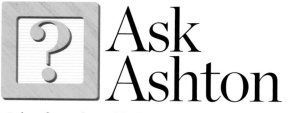

Ask Ashton

Is it safe to take probiotics when I'm pregnant?
—Scarlett K., Honolulu, HI

While there haven't been any studies showing that probiotics cause harm to moms or their babies, there aren't any studies proving a clear benefit, either. What we do know is that having a healthy community of gut microbes (what experts call your "microbiome") is very important for both maternal and infant health, helping with a wide range of pregnancy health issues, including gestational diabetes, and allergic diseases. See page 18 for more.

Is there anything I can eat during pregnancy that will help my kid get into Yale?
—Caitlin S., Los Angeles, CA

While starting a 529 savings plan is probably the best early move for your baby's educational future, focusing on a few key foods during pregnancy might help as well.

One study found that children whose mothers took supplements of cod liver oil during pregnancy and lactation scored higher on academic tests at age 4. (The magic nutrient was omega-3 fatty acids. In fact, moms who eat several weekly servings of fatty fish give birth to children with IQs five points higher than the spawn of fish-skippers, experts from the National Institutes of Health say.) Other studies found that children of women with the lowest percentage of iodine in their bloodstreams were in the lowest quartile for verbal IQ, reading accuracy, and reading comprehension. (To make sure you're getting enough iodine, toss the artisanal sea salt and use standard, iodine-fortified table salt—sparingly—to flavor your meals.)

Do I have to eat fish during my pregnancy, or can I just take a fish oil pill instead?
—Priyanka K., Oak Park, IL

Go fish! Fish provide fatty acids, minerals and vitamins that are essential for the growth of basically every cell in our bodies. Kids born from moms who eat fish regularly grow up to have higher childhood IQ scores, better fine-motor coordination, and stronger communication and social skills. But studies on fish oil pills have not found similar improvements in child development or health.

You mention folate is essential to a healthy pregnancy. What's your favorite source?
—Lisa W., Trenton, NJ

Folate (aka Folic Acid) is a type of water-soluble B vitamin. Foods that have it: Some grains and cereals are fortified with it, and it's also found in stuff you should be eating anyway, particularly leafy greens, as well as meats, veggies, fruits, and nuts. My favorite folate sources are romaine lettuce, broccoli, avocados, and strawberries.

Chapter

5

The
Third
Trimester
Diet

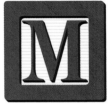**AYBE YOU'RE FREAKING OUT** a teensy bit about labor and delivery and would prefer to just stay pregnant rather than embark on that ordeal . . . or perhaps you feel impatient for baby to get here already—seriously, can your body support another pound of weight? The likely truth is that you're feeling both of these things—and much, much more. Your whole world has already changed and shifted through pregnancy, but you know that once your precious bundle arrives, nothing will ever be the same again—in the best way possible.

And while you're doing mental and emotional summersaults trying to figure out how the nursery will get finished in time—not to mention how much maternity leave you can really afford to take—baby is getting bigger and bigger. In fact, her weight will triple during these last few months, with her brain and lungs developing at lightning speed. And all that growth can end up making you more and more uncomfortable by the minute. It's understandable if your feet hurt, your legs hurt, your back hurts, your breasts hurt . . . and, well, does anything not hurt? Hint: If you have a partner, they so owe you a foot rub right now!

It would be awesome if I could tell you that eating certain things could make this final stretch of pregnancy breezier than a day at the beach (I can't), but the good news is that by eating a sensible diet and staying hydrated, you can keep yourself from feeling worse and keep some of the most dreaded third trimester pregnancy symptoms at bay.

What to Eat

Your general nutrition needs stay much the same as the first and second trimesters, but there are some areas you should focus on as your baby's nutritional needs increase during the final gestational growth spurt. Since biologically, your baby's nutritional needs are met before your own, you have to make sure that whatever food you eat is uber-nutritious and, at the same time, provides the extra calories that you need to keep yourself up and running at your peak.

You'll be gaining about a pound per week in this trimester, and ACOG recommends that to accommodate your speedily growing baby, you add about another 100 calories to your daily intake, or about 450 calories more than your pre-pregnancy/first trimester diet. And if you were overweight before you became pregnant, that number will likely be lower, since you won't need to gain as much over the course of your pregnancy. Of course, talk to your doctor and map out what your individual calorie intake should look like. Every mom-to-be's body is different and every pregnancy has its own specific needs. Keep that convo going with your OB or midwife.

Important word to the wise, though: Gaining too much weight during the third trimester increases the risk of the baby being born too large, and can increase your risk for pregnancy complications such as preeclampsia (extremely high blood pressure) and gestational diabetes; birth complications such as vaginal tears (um, ouch) and excess bleeding; and might increase

Fight Back with Food
Armed with these tips, you'll be a pregnancy symptom ninja!

The Problem:
Heartburn
You might not be able to avoid it entirely, but by making sure to eat small amounts through the day—and by finishing dinner or dessert three hours before bedtime —you can minimize its effects.

The Problem:
Hemorrhoids
Nom on plenty of fiber—it'll help keep things moving through your digestive system so you can avoid painful backups (and their horrible side effects!).

The Problem:
Swollen Legs
Avoid salty foods and drink plenty of water! Strange but true: Drinking more water actually helps nix water retention.

The Problem:
Leg Cramps
Ouch! These can be debilitating. Make sure you're getting plenty of potassium—bananas are a good and easy source. You'll be back to prenatal yoga in no time.

the need for a Caesarean section. Also, it's harder for you to lose the pregnancy weight afterward, which can put you at risk for obesity and complications during future pregnancies. So make sure to check in with your doctor.

Third trimester nutrition focus: During this last stretch, your baby's brain grows rapidly. The omega-3 DHA is especially important for brain and vision development throughout pregnancy and during nursing—yes, there are even DHA-enriched formulas you can buy! Check our Omega-3 guides on pages 14 and 70.

You should be getting at least 2 servings a week. If that isn't possible because you don't like fish or are vegetarian, you can take a supplement that contains at least 300 milligrams of DHA (vegetarian formulas are available)—but of course, discuss any supplements with your doctor before taking them.

The omega-3 in flax, walnuts, and chia seeds is a different form, known as ALA. There is some evidence that the body converts ALA to DHA in the body, so although those options aren't the best sources, they may still make smart choices, especially for vegetarians.

Your baby's skeletal system is making leaps and bounds of progress during the third trimester, so your calcium intake is crucial—make sure you're getting that 1,000 milligrams daily that ACOG recommends, because you'll be gearing up to produce breast milk.

Best calcium sources include milk—cow's, almond, soy, and most other plant milks, as long as they're fortified with calcium as well as vitamin D to enhance absorption.

Vegan sources include figs, almonds, and sesame seeds as well as dark green leafies: kale, collard greens and spinach; but this calcium is not as well absorbed as that found in dairy and other sources.

B-vitamins are essential nutrients—but did you know that there are eight B vitamins, including B 12 and B 6, which are required for proper blood cell formation and neurological function? Your body can't make them on its own, so getting them from food is vital.

Focus on real, not processed, food—100 percent whole grains, colorful fruits and veggies, nuts, legumes, extra-lean meats, and fatty fish—and you'll easily meet your need for these vitamins. Chickpeas also are an optimal source, along with peanut butter, and fortified whole-grain cereals.

Sample Daily Menu / Third Trimester

Breakfast

Protein Pancakes 1 medium banana, mashed + 2 eggs, whisked + 2 tbsp ground flaxseed + ½ cup oat flour. Mix and pan-fry in 1 tbsp coconut oil (serves 2)

Green Smoothie ¼ cup silken tofu, 2 kale leaves, ½ frozen banana, 1 cup unsweetened almond milk, 2 tbsp chia seeds

737 calories
31 g fat (13 g saturated)
151 mg sodium
21 g fiber
18 g sugar

Snack 1

Cashews, 3 tbsp

245 calories
19.5 g fat (3.7 g saturated)
271 mg sodium
12 g fiber
2 g sugar

Lunch

Grilled Chicken Salad Combine 12 oz cooked chicken with 1 bag prewashed arugula, ¼ cup dried cranberries, ¼ cup crumbled goat cheese, ¼ cup walnuts, vinaigrette, and salt and pepper to taste

100-calorie pack of store-bought guacamole and 2 crispbread crackers

150 calories
10 g fat (8.3 g saturated)
547 mg sodium
16.1 g fiber
4.6 g sugar

Snack 2

1 Low Fat String Cheese

½ cup celery topped with: 2 tablespoons peanut butter and 1 tablespoon raisins

547 calories
34.4 g fat (8.3 g saturated)
547 mg sodium
16.1 g fiber
4.6 g sugar

Dinner

Tuna burger on whole grain English muffin, toasted, with Romaine lettuce, sliced tomato, sliced red onion, 1 tsp olive-oil-based mayo

Kale salad with 3 cups chopped kale, 1 tsp extra-virgin olive oil, lemon juice, and 2 Tbsp sunflower seeds

417 calories
23 g fat (3 g saturated)
414 mg sodium
8 g fiber
3 g sugar

GRAND TOTAL = 2,257 calories / 128.9 g fat (31.2 g saturated fat) / 1,696 mg sodium / 60.6 g fiber / 36 g sugar

WIN THE DINNER WAR— BEFORE IT STARTS

Haven't even held your tiny baby in your arms and already nervous about getting him to eat his vegetables? Great news: You can take steps right now to tilt the odds of success in your favor. Studies have shown that babies who are exposed to vegetables in utero (yup, he can taste what you're eating through the amniotic fluid!) are more likely to develop a preference for them when they begin to eat solids.

Here's how it works: Flavors from your diet are also transmitted through your breast milk. One study published in *Pediatrics* showed that 4- to 8-month-olds whose nursing moms ate green beans accepted the vegetable more readily and ate three times more of them than did babies who were not so exposed. Your baby can even learn to like super healthy kale and greens if you eat them now on a regular basis.

Unfortunately, the same holds true for cookies, chips, and other no-nutrient snacks: Recent research discovered that when pregnant rats ate diets high in sugar and fat, their babies were born less sensitive to opioids, chemicals released by the brain when foods high in fat and sugar are eaten. That suggests children born with a tolerance for junk food may need to eat more of it to get the "feel good" response that causes other children to stop eating. And, well, that can lead to a host of health problems down the road.

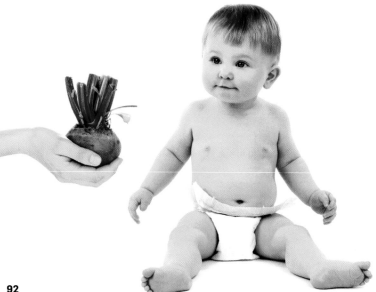

More Smart Snacks

To score the extra 450 calories you need to add on top of your first-trimester diet, work in three of these snacks a day—they average out to about 150 calories each. The snacks listed here contain mom- and baby-healthy nutrients such as calcium, fiber and protein; disease-fighting antioxidants; good fats; and even chocolate! Mix and match away:

¼ cup honey-roasted peanuts
= 150 calories

8 ounces 100% pomegranate juice
= 160 calories

1 cup lentil soup
= 140 calories

1 kiwi and 1 ounce string cheese
= 120 calories

1 cup nonfat yogurt mixed with 1 teaspoon wheat germ and
1 teaspoon ground flax seed
= 160 calories

3 Medjool dates
= 170 calories

1 cup low-fat chocolate milk
= 160 calories

1 ounce dark chocolate
= 140 calories

1 apple with 1 tablespoon nut butter (almond, cashew, peanut)
= 170 calories

1 cup red and yellow bell pepper strips with
3 tablespoons hummus or baba ghanoush
= 160 calories

1 hard-boiled egg with 1 cup tomato or vegetable juice
= 135 calories

1 cup chocolate frozen yogurt drizzled with 1 teaspoon chocolate syrup
= 140 calories

6 Ways to Add 450 Calories to Your Diet

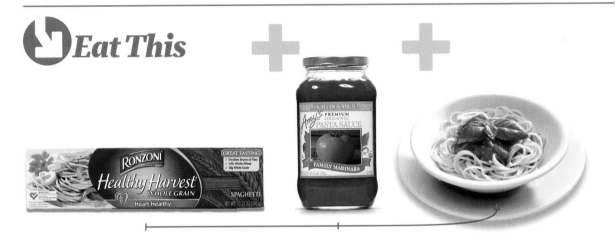

Ronzoni Healthy Harvest Whole Grain Spaghetti topped with ½ cup Amy's Light in Sodium Organic Family Marinara

260 calories
6 g fat (0.5 g saturated)
20 mg sodium
5 g carbohydrates
3 g sugar

When a craving for Italian hits, choose whole-grain pastas for an extra hit of fiber and top it with nutrient-rich marinara for a homemade meal that leaves room for more snacking.

OK, by now, you know the drill: In the third trimester, you're adding roughly 450 calories to your usual diet—aka your pre-pregnancy or first trimester diet. (If you're carrying twins, make it 500!) You want to make sure these are quality, nutrient-dense calories that will give your baby those essentials, and give you enough energy to keep ruling at everything you do—not tons of unhealthy fats.

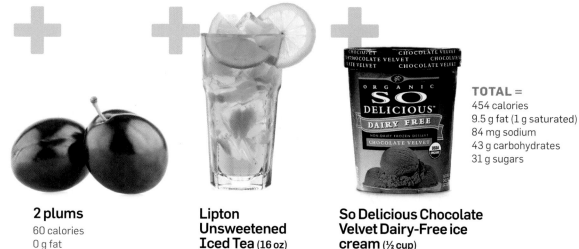

TOTAL =
454 calories
9.5 g fat (1 g saturated)
84 mg sodium
43 g carbohydrates
31 g sugars

2 plums
60 calories
0 g fat
0 mg sodium
14 g carbohydrates
14g sugars

Lipton Unsweetened Iced Tea (16 oz)
4 calories
0 g fat
14 mg sodium
1 g carbohydrates
0 g sugars

So Delicious Chocolate Velvet Dairy-Free ice cream (½ cup)
130 calories
3.5 g fat (0.5 g saturated)
50 sodium
23 carbohydrates
14 g sugars

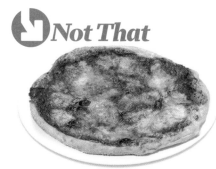

Not That

Uno Pizzeria & Grill Margherita Flatbread Artisan Crust Pizza (½ pie)
445 calories
14.5 g fat (7.5 g saturated)
750 mg sodium
47 carbohydrates
3.5 sugars

You'd think this simple flatbread pizza would be a healthy choice— but it's loaded with saturated fats and sodium.

⟲ *Eat This*

Bunch of red grapes
(10 grapes)

34 calories
0 g fat
1 mg sodium
9 g carbohydrates
8 g sugars

+

Two slices Nature's Own Double Fiber Wheat with 2 slices Kraft Singles 2% Milk Sharp Cheddar

290 calories
8 g fat (3 g saturated)
840 mg sodium
13 g carbohydrates
16 g protein

+

Kashi Layered Granola Bar Peanutty Dark Chocolate

130 calories
4.5 g fat (1 g saturated)
80 mg sodium
20 g carbohydrates
7 g sugars

TOTAL=
454 calories
12.5 g fat (4 g saturated)
921 sodium
41 g carbohydrates
31 sugars

A cheesy sandwich at home, surrounded by some healthy snacks, will always prove better than something coming at you through the window of your car.

⟲ *Not That*

McDonald's Bacon McDouble

440 calories
22 g fat (10 g saturated)
1,110 mg sodium
35 g carbohydrates
7 g sugars

Here's proof that coutning calories isn't all there is to eating thoughtfully. Although this sandwich has about 450 calories, it's also got 22 grams of fat, the equivalent of squirting three servings of Cheez Whiz into your belly.

Eat This

Jamba Juice 16-oz Strawberry Whirl Smoothie

210 calories
0 g fat
20 mg sodium
53 g carbohydrates
45 g sugars

½ cup mixed raspberries and blackberries

31 calories
0.5 g fat (0 g saturated)
0 mg sodium
3 g carbohydrates
3 g sugars

SeaPak Salmon Burger on a Martin's 100% Whole Wheat Potato roll
(with lettuce, tomato, onion)

223 calories,
6 g fat (1 g saturated)
521 mg sodium
18 g carbohydrates
5 g sugars

TOTAL =
464 calories
6.5 g fat (1 saturated)
541 mg sodium
74 g carbohydrates
53 g sugars

Go small on the smoothie to save room for some amazingly healthy fish and fiber-rich berries later on.

Not That

Jamba Juice 16 oz Chocolate Moo'd Smoothie

430 calories
4 g fat (2 g saturated)
270 mg sodium
86 g carbohydrates
77 g sugars

Holy cow, indeed. This smoothie is basically just a cup of chocolate fro-yo. Even in the smallest size, it's not doing you any favors.

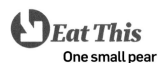
Eat This

One small pear

86 calories
0 g fat
1 mg sodium
23 g carbohydrates
15 g sugars

Panera Bread Full Strawberry Poppyseed & Chicken Signature Salad

350 calories
13 g fat (1.5 g saturated)
290 mg sodium
9 g carbohydrates
10 g sugars

8 baby carrots

28 calories
0 g fat
62 mg sodium
4 g carbohydrates
4 g sugars

TOTAL =
464 calories
13 g fat (1.5 g saturated)
353 mg sodium
35 carbohydrates
29 sugars

Want crunch? You can have a ton of it if you make smart choices. Side note? Baby carrots are a great grab-and-go snack for your handbag.

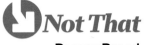
Not That

Panera Bread Apple Crunch Muffin

450 calories
12 g fat (2.5 g saturated)
30 mg sodium
0 g carbohydrates
49 g sugars

With more sugar than two Snickers bars, this muffin is more crash than crunch.

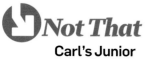Eat This

Applegate Organics Organic Chicken Strips,
served hot (3 pieces)

170 calories
8 g fat (1 g saturated)
350 mg sodium
12 carbohydrates
1 g sugars

Cascadian Farms Shoe String French Fries

110 calories
5 g fat (1 g saturated)
10 mg sodium
17 g carbohydrates
1 sugars

Apple

53 calories
0.1 g fat,
(0 g saturated)
1 mg sodium
10 g carbohydrates
10 g sugars

2 Newman's Own Newman-O's Chocolate Crème Filled Chocolate Cookies

110 calories
5 g fat (2 g saturated)
95 mg sodium
18 g carbohydrates
9 g sugars

TOTAL =
443 calories
18.1 g fat (4 g saturated)
456 mg sodium
57 g carbohydrates
21 sugars

Bake up some fries at home and you'll be able to add in some lean protein, fresh fruit and even cookies later on.

Not That

Carl's Junior CrissCut Fries
(side order)

450 calories
29 g fat (5 g saturated)
900 mg sodium
42 g carbohydrates
0 g sugars

Your baby is literally being made out of the foods and nutrients you consume. So why eat a side order with 900 grams of salt?

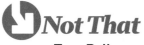

Eat This

Amy's Black Beans & Tomatoes Breakfast Burrito

270 calories
8 g fat,
(1 g saturated)
540 mg sodium
38 g carbohydrates
3 g sugars

½ cup mixed raspberries and blackberries

31 calories
0.5 g fat,
(0 g saturated)
0 mg sodium
3g carbohydrates
3g sugars

Evolution Fresh Organic Sweet Greens and Ginger

53 calories
0 g fat
169 mg sodium
12 g carbohydrates
10 g sugars

Stonyfield Oikos Organic Greek Yogurt Honey 0%

120 calories
0 g fat
75 mg sodium
26 g carbohydrates
17 g sugars

TOTAL =
474 calories
8.5 g fat (1 g saturated)
784 mg sodium
89 g carbohydrates
23 g sugars

A burrito for breakfast is tasty and convenient, and with this one, you can round out your morning meal with fresh fruit, juice, and a calcium-packed Greek yogurt.

Not That

Taco Bell Grilled Breakfast Burrito–Country

440 calories
34 g fat (7 g saturated)
930 mg sodium
45 g carbohydrates
5g sugars

It's the gravy and the nitrite-rich sausage that take this burrito from hero to zero.

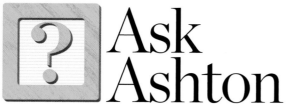

Ask Ashton

True or false: Pregnancy cravings mean you're low on the nutrients (like salt or iron) in the foods you crave (like fries and a burger!).
—Zoe B., Portland, OR

False. Craving a certain food during pregnancy—an iron-rich, juicy burger, say—does not mean your body is low in particular nutrients. The cravings you get are most likely to mimic the ones you've had in the past, especially when you were PMS-ing, according to a study published in the journal *Frontiers in Psychology*.

A baby only weighs about 8 pounds? What else is in my belly!?!
—Jazmin A., Mt. Dora, FL

It varies from woman to woman, but here's how those pounds might add up, according to the American College of Obstetricians and Gynecologists:

7.5 pounds: average baby's weight

7 pounds: extra stored protein, fat, and other nutrients

4 pounds: increased blood

4 pounds: increased body fluids

2 pounds: breast growth

2 pounds: growth of the uterus

2 pounds: amniotic fluid

1.5 pounds: the placenta

Is it true that a mani-pedi can actually harm pregnant women?
—Sofia H., White Plains, NY

It's tempting to hit the salon for a pretty, long-lasting pick-me-up, but hold it: The compounds in gel formulas are potentially toxic to you and baby. Gel polish won't seep into the nail itself, but it could be absorbed through the nail bed. To keep yourself and your peanut safe, opt for a regular mani and choose a polish that's free of dibutyl phthalate, or DBP, toluene, and formaldehyde. When it's time to dry your digits, opt for a fan with the UV light turned off; extra UV exposure is never good, whether you're preggers or not.

I've been pretty turned on during this pregnancy. How can I help my husband catch up?
—Brianna C., Palo Alto, CA

Encourage him to eat more foods that have been shown particularly effective at flattening the male belly and turbocharging the little man in the middle. "Spinach is rich in magnesium, a mineral that decreases inflammation in blood vessels, increasing blood flow," explains Cassie Bjork, RD, LD of Healthy Simple Life. And when it comes to a man, blood flow is everything. "Increased blood flow drives blood to the extremities, which can increase arousal and make sex more pleasurable," says psychotherapist Tammy Nelson, Ph.D. Spinach is also rich in folate, which increases blood flow to the nether regions, helping to protect your guy against age-related sexual issues.

Chapter

6

Eat This, Not That!

At Your Favorite Restaurants

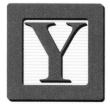

OU WOULDN'T LET A CLOWN BABYSIT your child. So why would let you one feed her?

That's a riddle I ask my patients when we discuss the perils—and pleasures—of eating out when pregnant. They think I'm about to deny them McDonald's, assuming fast food is off-limits. On the contrary, I tell them: You can enjoy McDonalds, or Denny's, or most fast food joints or sit-down restaurants. I just want to make sure *you're* the one deciding what to buy there, instead of the food marketers who just want your money.

This chapter will help you do just that.

Order Right, Every Time

Without a book like this, it's nearly impossible to make the right choice. That's because the people selling you food don't have your best interests in mind. Instead, the people selling you food are trying to—you guessed it—sell you food. And a lot of it. For them, it pays to sell us more for less—even if that "bargain" isn't great for baby. (Or for you, or Dad, for that matter.)

Here's a quick story that illustrates why.

Let's say you go to your local JCPenney to buy a maternity bathing suit. While you're there, you see a cool T-shirt that you just gotta have. Imagine each one costs the manufacturer

about the same to make, and each one is priced similarly, at about 30 bucks. You, however, have only $50 in your purse.

But, ooh, there's a sale! Buy one, get the other at 30 percent off! You could buy them both. You've essentially super-sized your order—and got a bargain.

What does this little tale have to do with your baby? It's simple: When we go into a restaurant, we use the same "shopping" thought process that we do when we hit the department store. But the results are wildly different. Because you're not buying clothes. You're buying calories, sodium and fat.

And too much of those can be very bad for your baby.

The Ground Rules

In order to make sure you order right, every time, the team at Eat This, Not That! combed more than 100 menus and analyzed the ingredients to find dishes that are low in sodium, reasonable in calories and full of healthy fats. The "Not Thats" listed are dishes that are, in comparison, less healthy.

For each category, you'll also get some ground rules, so you can make the right choice no matter where you are. In general, whether you're eating out or at home, it's prudent to ask:

- **Where's my protein?**
- **Where's my fiber?**
- **Where's my healthy fat?**

And I'd add one more, if you're at a restaurant:

- **Do I need this carb?**
  Like, do I *really* need this carb?

I know you really *want* that carb. But limiting your carb intake is the easiest way to control your weight during pregnancy. Your goal should be to find a meal that consists mainly of lean proteins, fruits and vegetables—like the ones in this chapter. (Hey, cheer up: Veggies are carbs!)

I limit carbs often and never leave hungry. For example, my daughter plays competitive ice hockey, and there are few places unhealthier than the food bar at an ice rink. Once, we were at a tournament, and I scanned the menu and told my son what I wanted: "Meatball sub with no bread."

When the order was ready, the server, clearly amused, decided to have some fun: "Meatball sub!" she yelled. "Just balls!" It's become a family joke, for when I order healthy: Just balls. But my point is, you can Eat This, Not That! anywhere. Read on to find out how.

3 Ways to Slim Down Your Order

Order Sauce on the Side
Same with dressing. And then use half of what they give you, or use it sparingly. Just the act of pouring it on yourself makes you aware of how much you're eating.

Ask for Two Containers
In your later stages, you'll have a smaller stomach capacity. Split your meal in two, and you won't eat more than you need.

Eat Before You Eat
Before you hit the restaurant for dinner, order an appetizer of a broth-based soup. Even an apple can reduce total calorie intake over the course of the meal by up to 20 percent, according to a series of "Volumetrics" studies at Penn State.

You're Craving a Burger

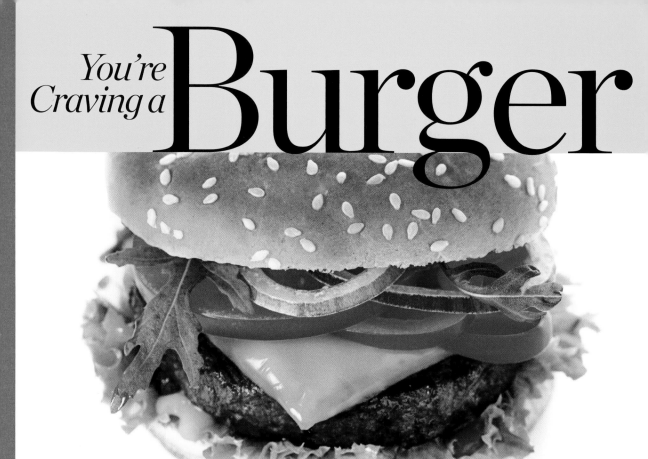

Burgers are an American birthright. And you're going to have a baby. So indulge once in a while! Topped with lettuce, tomato, onions, cheese, and a whole wheat bun, a hamburger can be a high-protein treat and an amazing source of baby-building iron. Just make sure the meat is fully cooked. Rare or undercooked meat could lead to a harmful infection with a very scary name (toxoplasmosis). Order your patty well-done.

PICK A PATTY
Let's get to the meat of the matter.

GROUND BEEF
It's an old wives' tale that pregnant women crave meat when their bodies need iron, but ground beef is, in fact, an excellent source of iron, mood-boosting B-vitamins, and selenium, which has been shown to reduce the risk of preeclampsia, a complication caused by high blood pressure. Eat it.

CHICKEN
With less cholesterol than ground beef, a chicken patty is my favorite go-to protein for ladies with babies—especially if it's grilled simply. Order yours fried or breaded, however, and you're adding a delicious crunch—but extra fat. Save those for occasional cheats.

TURKEY
Turkey has many of the same health benefits of ground beef—stock your fridge with some. But if you're eating out, be warned: Ground turkey meat dries out faster than beef, so restaurants often pack it with extra fat to keep it juicy. Ask your server or chef what they do.

VEGGIE
Suddenly cool—after years of tasting like hockey pucks—veggie burgers are loaded with healthy fiber and pack a lot less fat than meaty options. If the restaurant makes its own patties, they're likely to contain fewer preservatives, too.

GO FOR GRASS FED

Just as what you eat affects your baby, what a cow eats affects its meat. When you can, go for grass-fed beef. It contains fewer calories, and is packed with more omega-3s than even salmon! The all-natural chains below offer grass-fed varieties, and might be coming to a city near you:

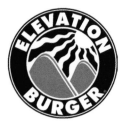
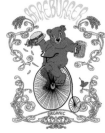
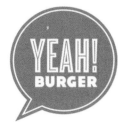
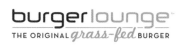

CHECK OUT THESE BUNS
Get a handle on our top four burger breads—well, top three.

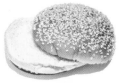

SESAME BUN
Your friends may tell you that sesame seeds aren't safe during pregnancy, but there's no scientific evidence of that—plus, sesame seeds can be a great source of bone-building calcium!

WHOLE WHEAT BUN
Always ask to swap a white bun for the whole wheat variety. The added fiber will keep you feeling full and help you beat bloat after downing a big burger.

SOURDOUGH BUN
Not only is the slightly tangy taste of the bread delish, but it packs some super benefits, too. The longer fermentation process of making sourdough bread actually makes it easier for your body to absorb all of the healthy folic acid, iron, zinc, and other nutrients it contains.

LETTUCE WRAP
While iceberg lettuce is mainly just water, the bunless route is a great idea if you're experiencing gestational diabetes and the only other option is a simple, nutritionally empty white bun.

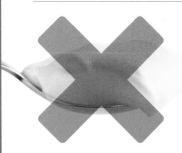

SAY NO TO THIS MAYO

If you think "a sandwich just isn't a sandwich" without mayo, don't worry: Store-bought brands are OK to eat. The processing kills off any raw-egg food-borne illnesses. The same can't be said for homemade mayos. Ask your server for the store-bought stuff.

TOP TOPPINGS Load up on these healthy extras.

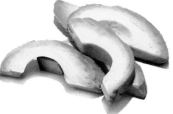

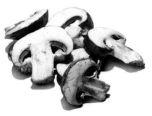

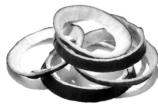

Avocado

Avocados are packed with good fats (think, the kind that give your hair extra shine!) and also boast a ton of folate, potassium, and vitamin B6, which can help beat morning sickness.

Mushrooms

Add a bit of sunshine to your burger with mushrooms, one of the only non-animal sources of vitamin D. The nutrient helps your body absorb calcium, and many women don't get enough.

Raw Onions

Want to beat the flu while you're pregnant? Onions have been shown to boost your immune system and can also add a fiber boost to your burger. Just remember to pack some mints.

Other Decent Options

- Tomatoes (if in season)
- Lettuce (organic, if they have)
- Spinach (organic, if they have)
- Pickles
- Sauerkraut
- Fried Egg

EVIL ADD-ONS
Just say no to these nutrition hamburglers.

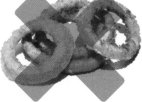

Chips

Yes, they're yummy. Yes, they add satisfying crunch. Nobody's arguing with you on those points, but they're simply not good for you. End. Of. Story.

Bacon

Recent studies link these crispy strips to a higher risk of cancer, unless they're uncured—not something you want to mess with.

Onion Rings

With all that extra breading and fat, these deep-fried rounds can barely be called a vegetable anymore.

Don't Be Fooled by:

- Blue cheese (often contains bad bacteria)
- Pre-washed spinach (wash it again!)
- Restaurant hot peppers (usually not maintained properly in the restaurant and full of bacteria!)

RULE #1: Indulge With

Eat This
McDonald's Cheeseburger
with small French Fries

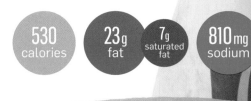

530 calories

23g fat

7g saturated fat

810mg sodium

17g protein

+

When it's
Burger Time,
PICK
THESE

Wendy's Junior Cheeseburger
With a name like that, how can you resist?

DQ Original Hamburger
Just a simple, straightforward classic.

Ted's Montana Grill's Skinny Dip Bison Burger
Bison is often leaner than beef.

You may be "eating for two," but that doesn't mean you need two patties for dinner. Order the smaller cheeseburger and you'll have room for fries!

But Skip These BURGER BOMBS

Hardee's and Carl's Jr. ½ Lb. Thickburger El Diablo
Eat this, and you get the fat and sodium equivalent of three Big Macs!

Ruby Tuesday's Portabella Crispy Onion Pretzel Cheeseburger
They add a healthy portabella mushroom, but use a salted pretzel as a bun.

Denny's Double Cheeseburger
Double trouble. That's the trans-fat equivalent of eight Whopper Jrs. piled high!

Not That!

McDonald's Double Quarter Pounder
with Cheese

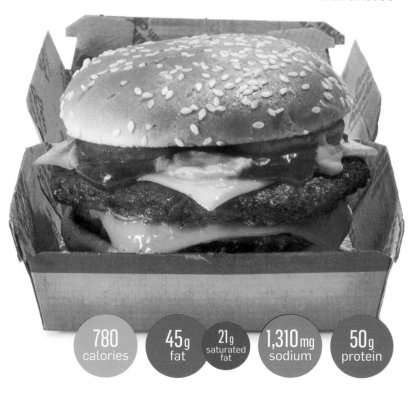

780 calories   **45g** fat   **21g** saturated fat   **1,310mg** sodium   **50g** protein

Don't make it a double. This may taste good going down, but it could make you gassy—and has more saturated fat than three and a half servings of Crisco!

RULE #2:
Look for Patty Substitutes

Veggie burgers are the mixtapes of the burger world: the best vegetables out there, mashed into one. Order right, and you'll find delicious varieties made with protein-packed beans (high in iron and zinc), chickpeas (high in vitamin B6 and choline) or quinoa (which has more protein than any other grain). And soy burgers are great, too: Each has more than 8 grams of protein, and is high in iron and vitamin B12.

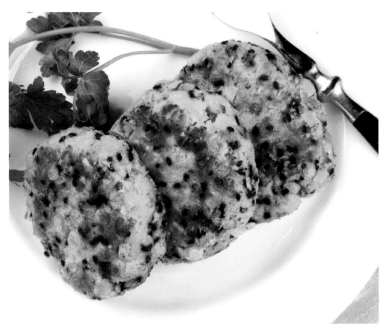

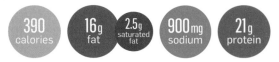

Eat This
Burger King Veggie Burger

It's rare to find a drive-thru veggie burger option, and this one shouldn't be missed. Get your burger buzz on without beefing up on fat and extra calories.

390 calories	16g fat	2.5g saturated fat	900mg sodium	21g protein

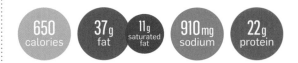

Not That!
Burger King Whopper

Over 200 calories more than the veggie burger, with only one gram more protein? It doesn't take a genius to figure out that this order isn't the smartest on the menu—for you, nor baby!

650 calories	37g fat	11g saturated fat	910mg sodium	22g protein

RULE #3:
Skip the Bun Sometimes

With apologies to Nicki Minaj, your baby doesn't want buns, hon. Most are empty carb vessels. You'd do better to replace them with a nutrient-heavy veggie like watercress, kale, or chard. You'll find delicious options at Bareburger (the Farmstead is wrapped in kale), Hardee's (try the low carb Thickburger), and even In-N-Out (try their "protein style" hamburger).

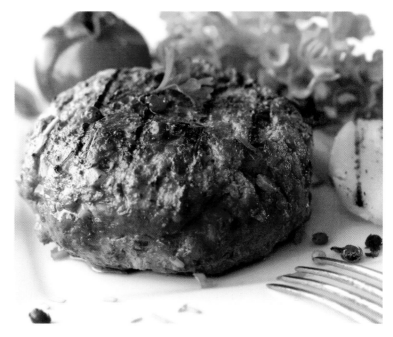

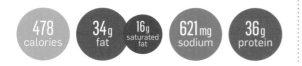

Eat This
Five Guys Bunless Burger (Double)
with Ketchup, Mustard, Pickles, Lettuce, and Tomato

You're obviously not going to Five Guys for a clean eating fest, but the chain does offer this awesome bunless option.

478 calories	34g fat	16g saturated fat	621mg sodium	36g protein

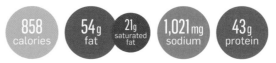

Not That!
Five Guys Hamburger
with Mayo, Ketchup, Pickles, Lettuce, and Tomato

Nearly double the calories and fat with very little added protein? The bun and added mayo might make baby cry even before she's born.

858 calories	54g fat	21g saturated fat	1,021mg sodium	43g protein

113

CREATE THE PERFECT BURGER

Dare to explore a world of burgers that no fast-food clown could ever imagine.

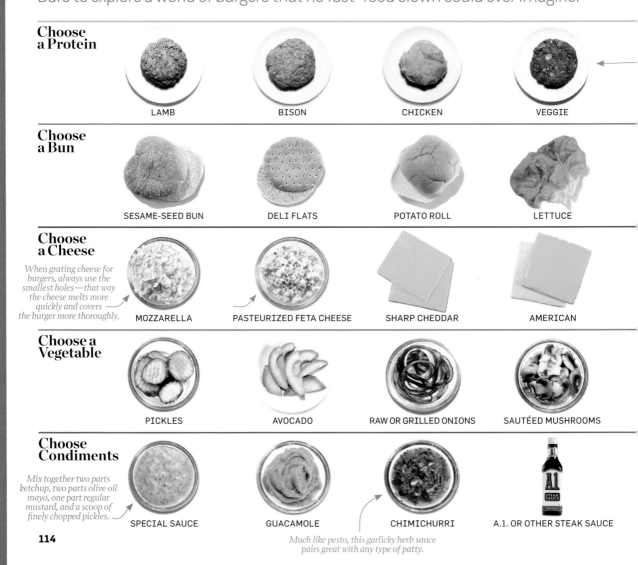

Choose a Protein

LAMB BISON CHICKEN VEGGIE

Choose a Bun

SESAME-SEED BUN DELI FLATS POTATO ROLL LETTUCE

Choose a Cheese

When grating cheese for burgers, always use the smallest holes—that way the cheese melts more quickly and covers the burger more thoroughly.

MOZZARELLA PASTEURIZED FETA CHEESE SHARP CHEDDAR AMERICAN

Choose a Vegetable

PICKLES AVOCADO RAW OR GRILLED ONIONS SAUTÉED MUSHROOMS

Choose Condiments

Mix together two parts ketchup, two parts olive oil mayo, one part regular mustard, and a scoop of finely chopped pickles.

SPECIAL SAUCE GUACAMOLE CHIMICHURRI A.1. OR OTHER STEAK SAUCE

Much like pesto, this garlicky herb sauce pairs great with any type of patty.

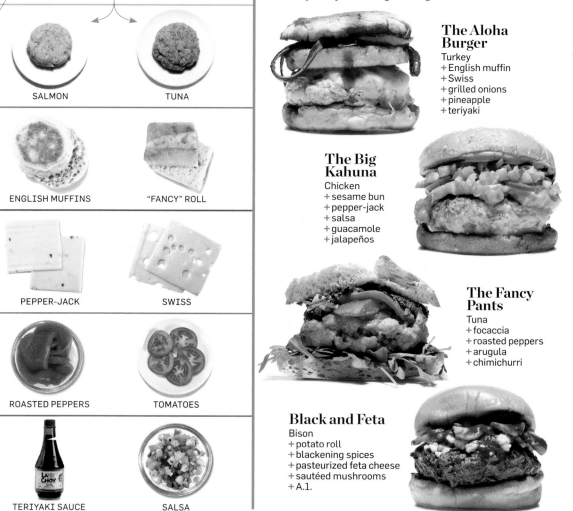

Make your own veggie patties by pureeing ½ pound mushrooms, 1 cup black beans, ¾ cup bread crumbs, 1 egg, and a few shakes of Worcestershire in a food processor.

To form tuna or salmon patties, chop 1 pound of meat very finely and combine with 1 egg, ½ cup bread crumbs, and any seasonings you want to add.

SALMON

TUNA

ENGLISH MUFFINS

"FANCY" ROLL

PEPPER-JACK

SWISS

ROASTED PEPPERS

TOMATOES

TERIYAKI SAUCE

SALSA

QUICK RECIPES

Choose your toppings carefully and cook your burger skillfully and you can't go wrong.

The Aloha Burger
Turkey
+English muffin
+Swiss
+grilled onions
+pineapple
+teriyaki

The Big Kahuna
Chicken
+sesame bun
+pepper-jack
+salsa
+guacamole
+jalapeños

The Fancy Pants
Tuna
+focaccia
+roasted peppers
+arugula
+chimichurri

Black and Feta
Bison
+potato roll
+blackening spices
+pasteurized feta cheese
+sautéed mushrooms
+A.1.

115

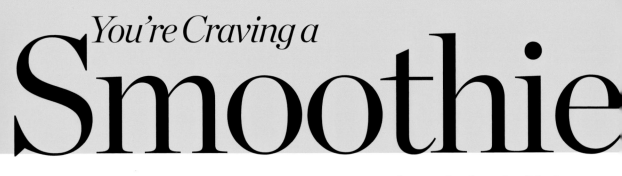

You're Craving a
Smoothie

It seems like the world's healthiest to-go option, right? Stick a bunch of fruit in a blender and . . . what could go wrong? The answer: Sugar. Some restaurant smoothies have more sugar than five Snickers bars, blended. Here's your guide to sipping smart.

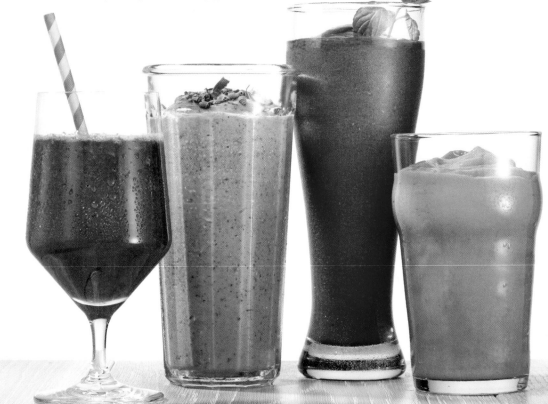

3 REASONS TO TREAT YO SELF

As if you needed another reason to order up a cup of yum!

1. YOU CAN'T KEEP ANYTHING ELSE DOWN

We all know morning sickness isn't limited to mornings—which can make it hard to get enough nutrients and calories to power your day. Because smoothies are already blended, they're easy on your stomach. Plus, sipping on something cold can actually help keep nausea at bay. Win-Win-Win!

2. YOU CAN'T MOVE ANYTHING OUT

Here's the thing. Constipation isn't cute. It's just not. It feels awful, and it's not exactly the thing you want to talk about during a night out with your girls. Still, a study out of Loyola Medicine showed that nearly 3 out of 4 women suffer from tummy troubles during pregnancy. One quick fix? Fiber—and smoothies are packed with the stuff.

3. YOU'RE TOO BUSY TO EVEN CHEW

Of course you need rest while you're expecting, but you also are probably still going to work, keeping up with your social life, running errands, and hitting up seemingly gazillions of doctor's appointments every week. A big sit-down lunch? Ain't nobody got time for that! So instead of skipping a meal (never do that!) or surviving off vending machine fare, grab a smoothie and take it with you.

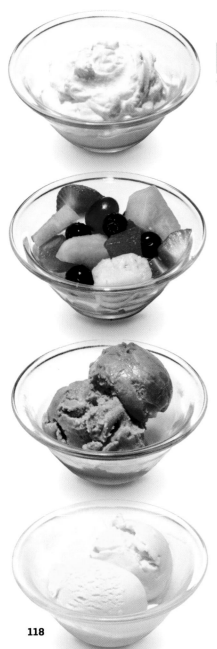

BACK TO BASE-ICS
What's the best for your belly? And your baby?

NON-DAIRY MILKS
Mixing your smoothie with dairy milk (I like 1%) is a great way to get protein, but 65% of Americans are lactose intolerant, thanks to a sugar that's hard to digest and causes bloating. That's why I recommend you make your smoothies with a plant- or nut-based milk like almond or cashew.

GREEK YOGURT
If your local shop whips up their fruit with a healthy dollop of Greek yogurt, both you and your tiny stowaway will get an energizing protein boost.

ALL FRUIT
The great thing here is that you know what you're getting—and what you're not (added chemicals and fat!). Just be sure to watch your portion size, since a massive serving of even natural sugars could cause you to crash during that important 4pm meeting!

FROZEN YOGURT
Here's a little truth bomb: Your average frozen yogurt probably isn't as fatty or as calorie-laden as ice cream (not much is!), but it's also lacking the super protein punch of its Greek yogurt cousin. Unless your smoothie shop uses non-fat froyo, ask if they can skip it.

ICE CREAM OR SHERBET
Some smoothies you get at restaurants and juice shops are actually little more than glorified milk shakes. All that added fat and sugar can add up. When ordering, make sure your smoothie isn't dessert.

BEST

WORST

SMOOTHIE ALL-STARS

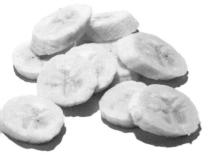

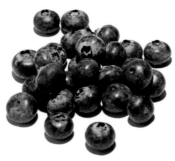

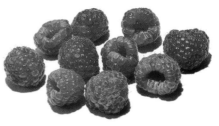

Bananas

Folic acid is key in preventing neural tube defects in your little one, and bananas are chock full of the stuff.

Blueberries

These colorful guys aren't just energizing, they're also packed with B vitamins that can help keep your moods swinging upward.

Raspberries

Just one cup of raspberries has roughly a third of the fiber you need in a day to keep things, ahem, moving along smoothly.

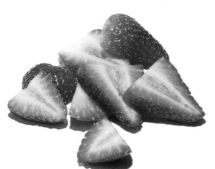

Strawberries

These berry patch favorites are relatively low in sugar, and boast a sky-high amount of immune-boosting vitamin C—ounce for ounce, even more than oranges!

Carrots

The natural sweetness of carrots plays well with all your other smoothie favorites. Plus, they contain tons of vitamin A, which is key in keeping your eyes sharp and helping to make sure baby's vision will be top-notch.

RULE #1: Beware of Mis

Eat This

**Red Mango
Strawberry
Sonata**
24 oz

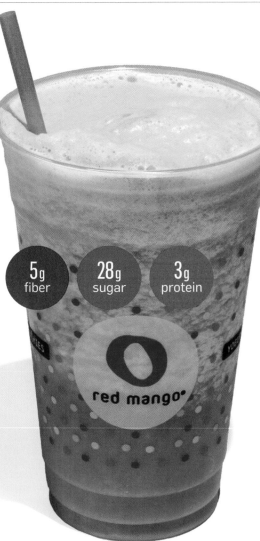

230 calories

1g fat

0g saturated fat

5g fiber

28g sugar

3g protein

With almost 100 fewer calories and more fiber than the smoothie on the right, this all-fruit pick will give you a steady stream of energy and keep you feeling full until your next meal.

**Enjoy
These
SMOOTH
MOVES**

Smoothie King Lean Strawberry Smoothie, 20 oz The simpler, the better when it comes to smoothies. This shake has only two ingredients: protein and strawberries.

Panera Bread Superfruit Power Smoothie with Ginseng, Small For a moderate 210 calories, this superfood smoothie boasts an impressive 14 grams of protein.

Juice Generation Green Guardian Smoothie, 20 oz Spinach, swiss chard, avocado, hemp seeds, chia seeds, flax seeds and strawberries make for a snack-sized 175 calories.

leading Menus

**Skip
These
BAD
BLENDS**

**Smoothie King
The Hulk
Strawberry,** 20 oz
Steer clear:
It's actually what
Smoothie King
calls a "weight
gain" drink,
made with butter
pecan ice cream
and a "weight
gain blend."

**Cold Stone
Strawberry
Mango, Love It,**
20 oz
Hate it. With
85 grams of
sugar, you'd be
drinking the
liquid equivalent of
four Kit Kat bars.

**Tropical
Smoothie Jetty
Punch**
This packs quite
a punch indeed:
It's got as
much sugar as
seven servings of
Lucky Charms.

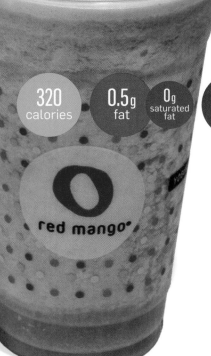

red mango°

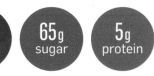

Not That!
**Red Mango
Strawberry
Energizer**
24 oz

320 calories	0.5g fat	0g saturated fat	4g fiber	65g sugar	5g protein

That "energizer"
feeling is the sugar
coursing through
your veins. Believe
it or not, this
super-sweet yogurt-
based smoothie is on
Red Mango's
"Body Balance" menu.
Just say no.

121

RULE #2:
Add Some Veggies When You Can

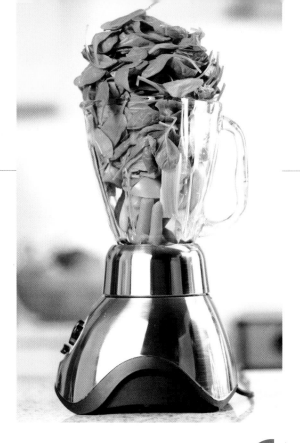

Opt for green smoothies—rather than green juices—whenever you can: Blenders preserve the satiating insoluble fiber that juicers press out. I love kale and watercress as a base, but spinach is especially powerful when it comes to controlling weight gain. In one Swedish study, 19 overweight women drank a mixture with five grams of spinach extract each morning. After three months, they reported fewer food cravings.

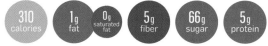

Eat This
Jamba Juice
Orange Carrot Karma 28 oz

We know you can't wait to look into your baby's eyes, but you also want to make sure they'll be healthy! The vitamin A in this carrot-infused blend will help protect those tiny peepers as they form in the second trimester.

310 calories	1g fat	0g saturated fat	5g fiber	66g sugar	5g protein

Not That!
Jamba Juice
Orange Dream Machine 28 oz

Made with both sherbet and nonfat frozen yogurt, it's no wonder this has almost double the sugar and calories—and only a tiny fraction of the fiber—of its counterpart.

590 calories	2g fat	1.5g saturated fat	1g fiber	120g sugar	12g protein

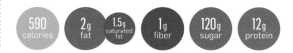

RULE #3:
Order the Right Chocolate

Ask your local smoothie shop to blend with raw cacao. It's packed with powerful antioxidants and boasts a surprisingly high amount of fiber. Paired with a portioned amount of honey, you'll find it as sweet and indulgent as a Hershey's, except it's actually good for you. Try the Chocolate Smoothie at Dig Inn for a taste.

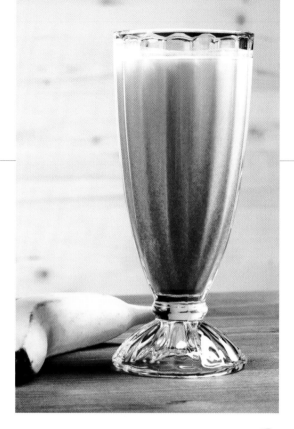

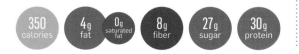

Eat This
Planet Smoothie Planet Pro Lite Cocoa & Banana 22 oz

With more protein than many burgers, this is a great go-to when you don't have time for a proper lunch. Added bonus? Bananas are great at calming nausea.

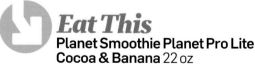

350 calories	4g fat	0g saturated fat	8g fiber	27g sugar	30g protein

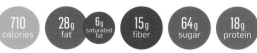

Not That!
Planet Smoothie PBJ 22 oz

This smoothie packs almost none of the nutritious benefits of a real peanut butter and jelly sandwich on whole wheat. Skip this goober of a smoothie.

710 calories	28g fat	6g saturated fat	15g fiber	64g sugar	18g protein

THE SMOOTHIE MATRIX

Get optimal nutrition with the press of a button.

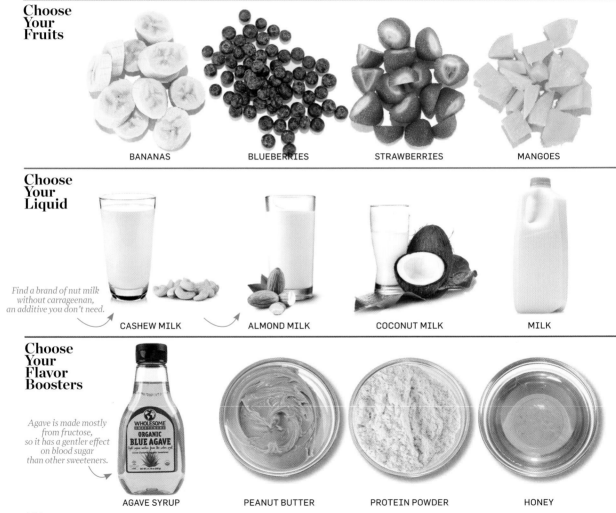

Choose Your Fruits

BANANAS   BLUEBERRIES   STRAWBERRIES   MANGOES

Choose Your Liquid

Find a brand of nut milk without carrageenan, an additive you don't need.

CASHEW MILK   ALMOND MILK   COCONUT MILK   MILK

Choose Your Flavor Boosters

Agave is made mostly from fructose, so it has a gentler effect on blood sugar than other sweeteners.

AGAVE SYRUP   PEANUT BUTTER   PROTEIN POWDER   HONEY

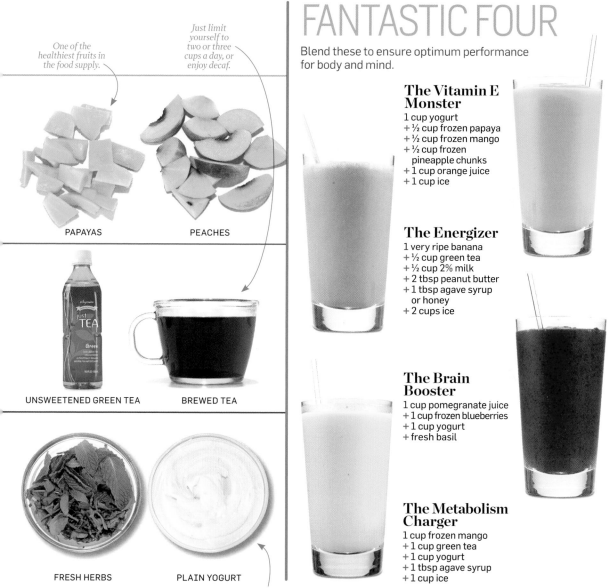

One of the healthiest fruits in the food supply.

Just limit yourself to two or three cups a day, or enjoy decaf.

PAPAYAS

PEACHES

UNSWEETENED GREEN TEA

BREWED TEA

FRESH HERBS

PLAIN YOGURT

As always, plain Greek yogurt like Fage and Oikos are best; just a cup of this stuff packs more than 15 grams of protein.

FANTASTIC FOUR

Blend these to ensure optimum performance for body and mind.

The Vitamin E Monster
1 cup yogurt
+ ½ cup frozen papaya
+ ½ cup frozen mango
+ ½ cup frozen pineapple chunks
+ 1 cup orange juice
+ 1 cup ice

The Energizer
1 very ripe banana
+ ½ cup green tea
+ ½ cup 2% milk
+ 2 tbsp peanut butter
+ 1 tbsp agave syrup or honey
+ 2 cups ice

The Brain Booster
1 cup pomegranate juice
+ 1 cup frozen blueberries
+ 1 cup yogurt
+ fresh basil

The Metabolism Charger
1 cup frozen mango
+ 1 cup green tea
+ 1 cup yogurt
+ 1 tbsp agave syrup
+ 1 cup ice

You're Craving Breakfast

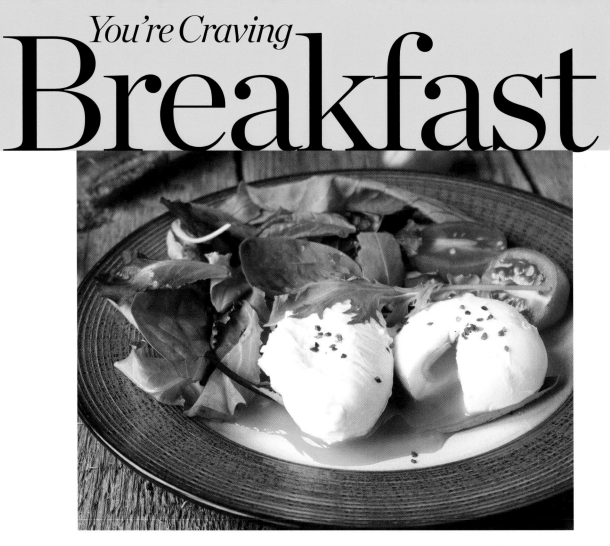

When you're sick in the morning, and are finally able to stomach something, there's nothing more comforting than, well, comfort food. The great news is that your morning favorites don't have to throw your whole day off track. Here's how to get things off to a healthy start.

ORDER RIGHT, EVERY TIME

These healthy hacks are an easy way to get the most from your meal.

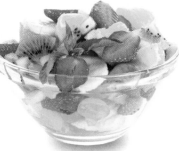

ASK FOR BUTTER ON THE SIDE

There's no need to eat your pancakes or toast dry, but adding it yourself allows you to control the portion—and know how much fat you're really adding to your meal.

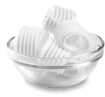

FILL UP ON FRUIT

If there's a fruit bowl on the menu, add it to your meal and eat it first. Better yet, add some atop plain oatmeal with some 1% milk for the perfect breakfast.

BANISH THE BAGEL

Did you know that one bagel has almost as many calories as four slices of bread? Go for fiber-rich whole wheat toast instead.

SUPER-CHARGE THAT OMELET

Cheese is delicious—and a great source of calcium—so get some in your omelette along with healthy veggies like bell peppers, spinach, and tomatoes. Pregnancy perfection!

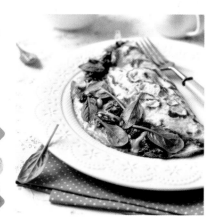

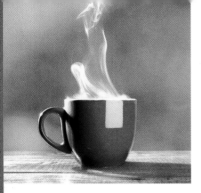

SIP SWAPS
Your morning drink shouldn't be an afterthought.

⟳ Drink This
Decaf coffee with milk
Even decaffeinated coffee has a tiny bit of caffeine, so you'll still get a pick-me-up—and the milk adds healthy bone-building calcium to an otherwise nutrient deficient part of your meal.

⟳ Or This
Black tea
Varieties like English Breakfast or Earl Grey have less caffeine than a cup of regular coffee, so you can safely have about three cups a day. Add some moo-juice for that creamy, calcium-boosted kick.

⟳ Not That
Sugary coffee drinks
One or two small cups (8 ounces each) of lightly-sugared black coffee per day are fine, but you'll have to give up your six-a-day Mocha Mega-Smoothie habit. Some have more than 1,500 grams of sugar!

⟳ Drink This
Seltzer with a splash of orange juice
This festive take on your morning sunshine will help you stay hydrated, which can ease a whole host of pregnancy-related ailments like headaches, cramps, and bloating.

⟳ Not That
A tall glass of orange juice
The mass-produced orange juice varieties that most restaurants serve lacks the nutrients of fresh squeezed—but even straight out of the juicer, this stuff will give you a big spike in blood sugar.

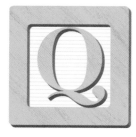

DOES IT MATTER HOW I ORDER MY EGGS?

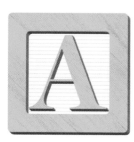

With about 6 grams of protein in each egg, these guys should be your breakfast BFFs—and knowing how to order them can actually make them even healthier. Poached eggs are the best option, since they're cooked in water and not fried. Scrambled can be a good choice, too—especially if you add in nutritious veggies like broccoli or spinach. Fried eggs are usually the least healthful option, but they're still a whole lot better for you than a buttery croissant!

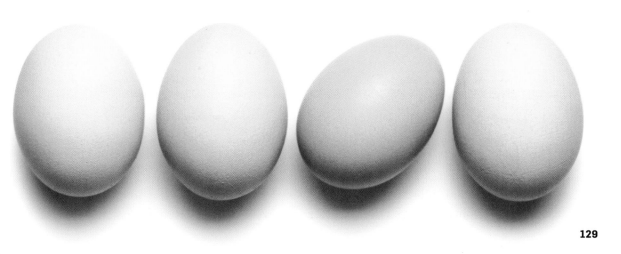

RULE #1: Egg Whites Do

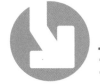

Eat This
IHOP Simple & Fit Vegetable Omelet with pre-cut fruit mix

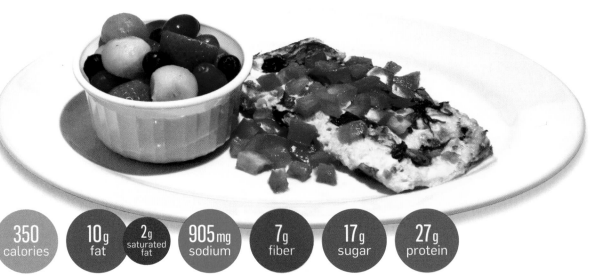

| 350 calories | 10g fat | 2g saturated fat | 905mg sodium | 7g fiber | 17g sugar | 27g protein |

Simple is the key here. You'll get iron, calcium, protein, and other pregnancy power-nutrients through the omelet and plenty of fiber through the fruit. No muss, no fuss, no bacon on the side.

Even Better Breakfasts

McDonald's Egg McMuffin
Yup, the classic. It's a staple Eat This, Not That! has approved for years. The yolk contains carotenoids, essential fatty acids, vitamins and minerals.

Dunkin' Donuts Egg and Cheese English Muffin Sandwich
With 12 grams of protein and less sodium than in years past, this is a Dunkin' Do.

Bob Evans Veggie Omelet
Cheers to this chain, which has been ranked a Not That! for years, but now offers this low-cholesterol option. You can also build your own omelet here.

Not Equal Healthy

Not That!
IHOP Harvest Grain 'N Nut Egg White Combo

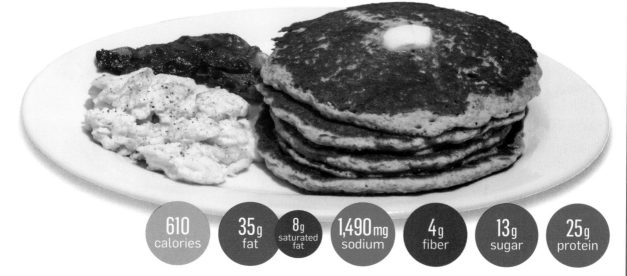

| 610 calories | 35g fat | 8g saturated fat | 1,490mg sodium | 4g fiber | 13g sugar | 25g protein |

From the name alone, you'd think egg whites would be the star of this meal, but they're not! Instead, you're getting carb-heavy pancakes and some unhealthy bacon along with a small portion of egg whites.

**Bob Evans
The Rise and Shine**
You'll wake up to 1,800 mg of sodium, nearly a day's worth before 9am. More like Rise and Swine.

**Dunkin' Donuts
Multigrain Bagel with Reduced Fat Strawberry Cream Cheese**
The "reduced fat" sounds healthy, but this breakfast is bogus, filled with refined carbs and low-grade fats.

**McDonald's
Steak, Egg & Cheese Bagel**
One sandwich has as much sodium as 16 Chicken McNuggets!

The Worst Ways to Start Your Morning

RULE #2:
Design Your Own Meal

If ever there was a time to be "that woman"—the one with the custom order—it's breakfast time. If the restaurant serves eggs, there's no reason why they can't make you two with a side order of whole wheat toast, unsweetened fruit, and a lean meat. But if you just have to have pancakes, check out the Eat This! below.

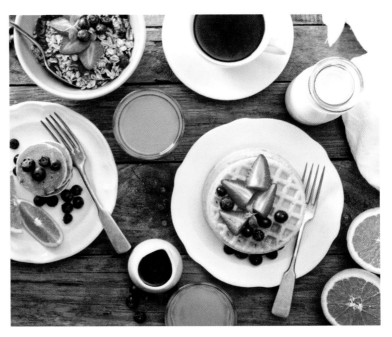

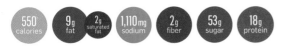

Eat This
Denny's Pancake Puppies
with a side of scrambled egg whites

No matter how you shake it, pancakes aren't a perfect breakfast pick. Still, if you order them as a side and get some protein-packed egg whites to go with them, it won't be an entire loss!

| 550 calories | 9g fat | 2g saturated fat | 1,110mg sodium | 2g fiber | 53g sugar | 18g protein |

Not That!
Fit Fare Banana Pecan Pancake Breakfast

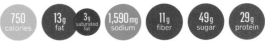

This option is marketed as being healthy, but all that bacon fat—not to mention the nitrites hiding in the crunchy strips—isn't good for you or baby. Order items a la carte if you want to avoid the bad stuff.

| 750 calories | 13g fat | 3g saturated fat | 1,590mg sodium | 11g fiber | 49g sugar | 29g protein |

RULE #3:
Scale Down the Sweet Stuff

It's OK to crave sweets while you're pregnant. It's another thing to order them for breakfast. IHOP has New York Cheesecake Pancakes. Perkins sells ones called Apple Pie. And Denny's Peanut Butter Cup Pancake Breakfast out-sweets them all, with more sugar than 5 servings of Edy's Ice Cream. Avoid them all and get something sweet, if you must—but make your main a protein.

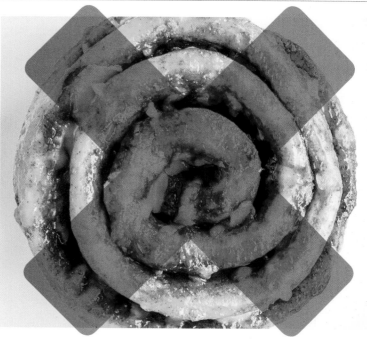

Eat This
Bob Evans Cherry Crepes

This is by no means a nutritional superstar. But for a once-in-a-while treat it's not too bad— especially since the cream cheese filling packs some protein and bone-building calcium.

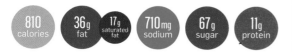

810 calories	36g fat	17g saturated fat	710mg sodium	67g sugar	11g protein

Not That!
Bob Evans Cherry Buttermilk Hotcakes

There's more sugar in this stack of pancakes than in three regular sized Hershey's bars— and the out-of-this-world sodium levels will leave you feeling heavy and bloated all day.

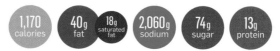

1,170 calories	40g fat	18g saturated fat	2,060g sodium	74g sugar	13g protein

133

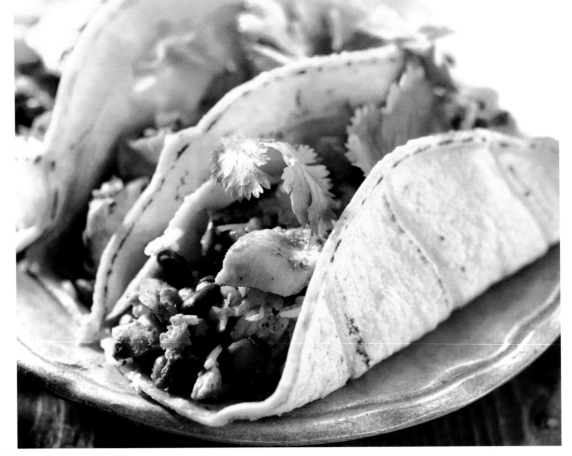

134

Obviously, mamacita's not having the margaritas, but pregnancy is no reason why you can't enjoy something south of the border. In fact, many traditional Mexican dishes contain healthy fats, calcium, and protein that your little one needs. Just be sure to limit the spicy options, heavy cheeses, and refried beans, unless you want to feel the (heart)burn.

ORDER RIGHT, EVERY TIME
Navigating the menu at your local cantina doesn't have to be tricky.

ASK ABOUT THE BEANS
If made with whole, all-natural beans, a fiberlicious bean burrito could be the healthiest thing on the menu—but if they're refried and cooked with lard, you'll be better off ordering chicken.

GET YOUR MOLE ON
This smoky sauce won't weigh you down the way sour cream will, and it's power-packed with flavor.

PASS THE PESCADO
Look for fish tacos or camarones—shrimp!—on the menu. They'll deliver a hefty dose of brain-building omega-3s to your baby.

KEEP IT SIMPLE
Anything listed on the menu as "supreme" is probably supremely loaded with unhealthy fats and salt that will make you feel puffy and bloated. Stay away!

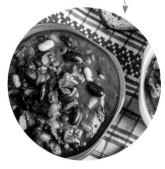

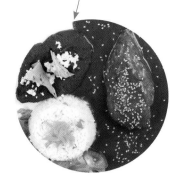

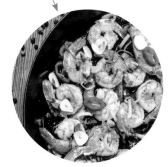

DIPPING DO'S AND DON'TS

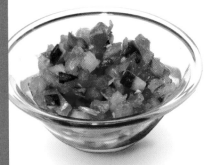

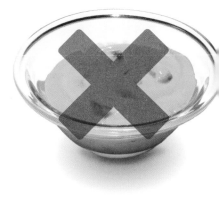

PICO DE GALLO

The fresh tomatoes in this festive salsa contain lycopene, a nutrient that some experts believe can prevent high blood pressure and hypertension during pregnancy.

GUACAMOLE

Guacamole may feel like an indulgence, but it's actually a pregnancy superfood! Not only can avocados help take the edge off the morning sickness blues, but they're also full of folate, which has been shown to protect against birth defects. Go ahead and dig in!

SOUR CREAM

One tablespoon of sour cream isn't going to throw you off track, but most restaurants are laying it on way thicker than that. Always make sure to order it on the side and use sparingly. It's delicious for sure, but nutritious it isn't!

QUESO

The high sodium content of queso dip, along with its crazy high fat content, isn't going to do your baby any favors. Skip out on the gooey orange stuff and opt for a fresher choice instead.

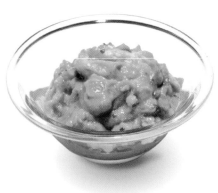

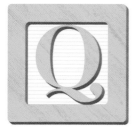

Q

IS IT SAFE TO EAT SPICY FOOD WHILE I'M PREGNANT?

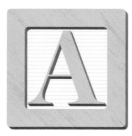

Yes! As long as picante flavors aren't giving you heartburn, it's 100 percent okay to get spicy. In fact, eating diverse types of food while you're pregnant will expose your baby to a wide variety of flavors while she's still in the womb, which experts say may make her less inclined to be a picky eater later on. Another bonus of adding a little heat to your meal? Spicy foods are excellent at clearing your sinuses and helping you breathe better. As for the rumor that these types of dishes can bring on labor? It's just that—a rumor, and nothing else!

RULE #1: Pick a Tortilla

Eat This

Chipotle Soft Corn Tortilla Tacos
with Steak, Cheese, Lettuce, and Fresh Tomato Salsa

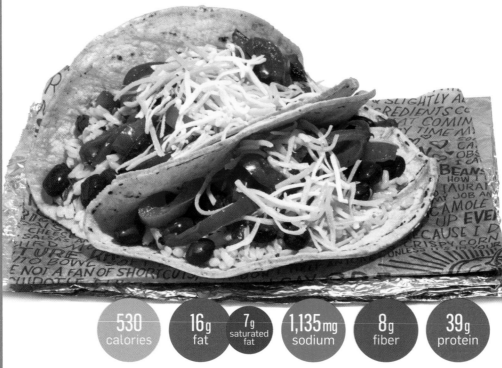

530 calories	16g fat	7g saturated fat	1,135mg sodium	8g fiber	39g protein

Say ¡Si! to These!

Baja Fresh Shrimp Americano Soft Taco
Enjoy one—not two—to keep the salt down.

Del Taco Turkey Taco (soft)
You get the benefits of lean turkey for only 170 calories.

Chipotle Chicken Bowl
Get one with brown rice, fajita vegetables, fresh tomato salsa, romaine lettuce and ½ serving of guac for the ultimate mex fest.

Your body uses iron to make extra blood for your little one, and steak delivers more than 20 percent of the amount you need in a day. Plus, this protein and fiber combo will fill you up without weighing you down with rice.

or Rice—not Both

¡No! ¡No! ¡No!

Baja Fresh Shrimp Fajitas with Flour Tortillas
Just one order has more than a day's worth of sodium!

Del Taco Flatbread Taco (Chicken)
The foamy breading adds needless calories—this has 150 more than the soft Turkey Taco.

Chipotle Carnitas Bowl
Order yours with white rice and the roasted chili-corn salsa, along with cheese and guacamole, and you have a burrito's-worth of carbs. Muy mal.

Not That!
Chipotle Burrito
with Steak, Black Beans, White Rice, Cheese, Sour Cream, and Roasted Chili-Corn Salsa

| 1,115 calories | 39.5 g fat | 15.5 g saturated fat | 2,165 mg sodium | 19 g fiber | 58.5 g protein |

The calorie count skyrockets when you've got two big starch items on your plate—in this case, a large flour tortilla and a heaping scoop of rice. Do your body and your baby a favor and go for one or the other—not both!

RULE #2:
If It Crunches, Don't Munch It

...because it's likely been fried. If you need a tortilla fix, do what Marisa Moore, RDN, does. "It could just be my love of anything with avocados, but in my eyes, few things beat a bowl of authentic tortilla soup," she says. "It's nourishing, comforting, and satisfying—but doesn't carry a lot of calories. It's perfect for a light meal or appetizer."

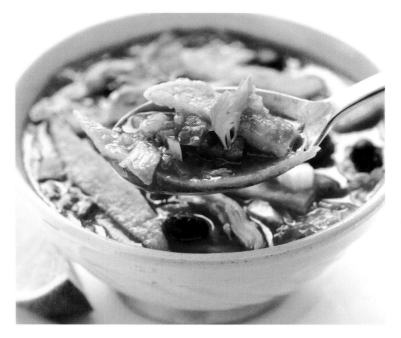

Eat This
Taco Bell Chicken Soft Tacos (2)

Soft tacos aren't just more authentic, they also contain less unhealthy fat than their crispier cousins, which get their crunch by being fried in oil.

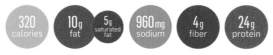

320 calories • 10g fat • 5g saturated fat • 960mg sodium • 4g fiber • 24g protein

Not That!
Taco Bell Crunchy Taco Supreme (2)

With double the fat and less protein, ordering these tacos might land you in Supreme court.

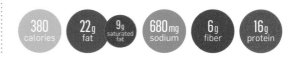

380 calories • 22g fat • 9g saturated fat • 680mg sodium • 6g fiber • 16g protein

RULE #3:
Watch Out for Sneaky Salads

Foolproof yourself against caloric ingredients by bowling. "When I'm at a Mexican restaurant, I like to keep it simple," recommends Isabel Smith, MS, RD, CDN. "I'll order an entree-size house salad in a bowl—not a taco shell—and ask my server to add beans, grilled chicken, avocado, and a light sprinkling of cheese. The black beans have soluble fiber that slows digestion, keeping me feeling fuller, longer."

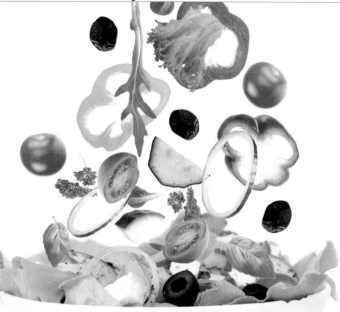

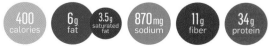

Eat This
On the Border Mango Chicken Salad
with Fat-Free Mango Citrus Dressing

Low in fats, high in fiber and protein? This salad will help keep your digestive system humming and give you plenty of energy to get the nursery put together (you know you've been putting it off!).

400 calories	6g fat	3.5g saturated fat	870mg sodium	11g fiber	34g protein

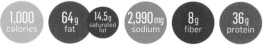

Not That!
On the Border Grande Taco Salad
Chicken Tinga with Smoked Jalapeño Vinaigrette

Clocking in at more than twice the calories and more than 10 times the fat, this salad is anything but healthy for you and your precious cargo. Blame the giant fried shell and the not-so-lean dressing.

1,000 calories	64g fat	14.5g saturated fat	2,990mg sodium	8g fiber	36g protein

You're Craving
A Sandwich

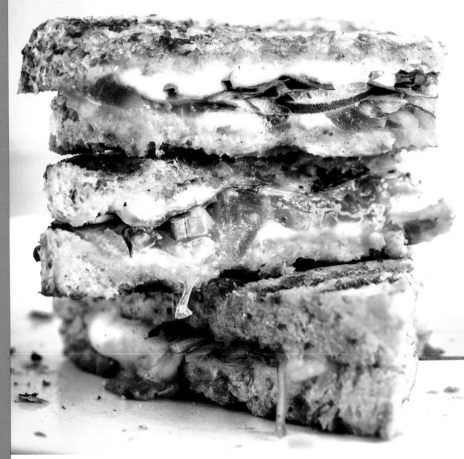

Perfect on a picnic, on-the-go, or in your lunchbag, the humble sandwich is the perfect way to work fiber, protein, and other important nutrients into your day, just as mom knew years ago. Now here's the bad news: If you're ordering one from a chain restaurant, mom's not the chef. Read on to discover how to order right.

THE GREAT BREAD BREAKDOWN

It's what's on the outside that counts.

#1 BEST

100% WHOLE GRAIN OR WHOLE WHEAT

Almost any type of bread can be made with whole wheat, which is made using the whole kernel of wheat, or whole grain, which could contain whole grains of any variety—including wheat, oats, spelt, or barley. You'll get a big fiber boost and feel fuller longer.

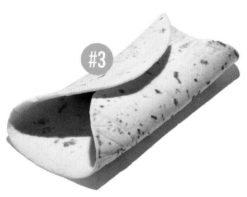

#3

WRAPS

Unless a wrap is whole wheat or whole grain, you're not doing yourself any favors by rolling your sandwich up in one. In fact, many have added fats to increase their flexibility.

#2

FOCACCIA

Since it often has cheese and oil baked right into it, getting your sandwich on focaccia can be the nutritional equivalent of wrapping your sandwich in a big slice of pizza.

CIABATTA

This Italian white bread is pillowy soft, but comes up short in terms of nutrients.

#5

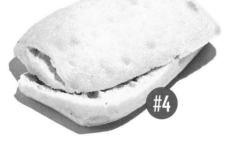

#4

FLATBREAD

Ounce for ounce, flatbreads may not be much healthier than other choices, but since there's typically less bread in a flatbread than in a roll or bun, they're often lower in calories.

143

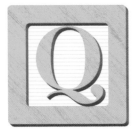

Q

CAN I EAT DELI MEATS?

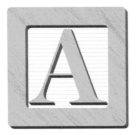

A

When you're pregnant, it's important to ALWAYS order deli meat sandwiches hot! Roughly 85 percent of illnesses from *Listeria*, a bacteria that can cause miscarriage, are caused by eating deli meats—and a recent study of three U.S. states showed that a whopping 70 percent of delis tested positive for *Listeria*. The good news is that this invisible, odorless bacteria can be killed if it's heated to a piping hot 165 degrees. Some women choose to give up deli meats altogether until baby arrives, but if you're not among them, just make sure to heat up those cold cuts before indulging.

Go ahead! But ONLY if you heat me up!

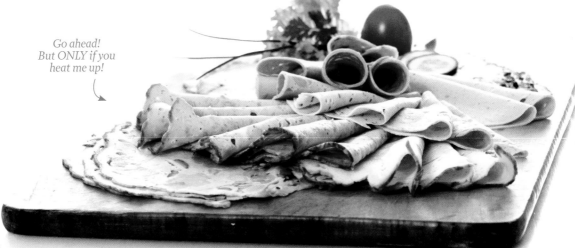

SAY CHEESE! AND HUMMUS

Don't want a hot sandwich? More and more restaurants are serving up delish meatless sandwiches that don't need to be heated up.

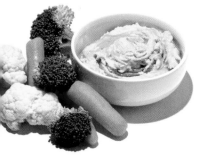

HUMMUS AND VEGGIES

With a perfect balance of protein, fiber, and healthy fats, this Mediterranean combo might indeed be a gift from the gods!

PORTOBELLO MUSHROOM

Not only are these mushrooms big on protein (who knew?!) but they also contain a good amount of thiamine, which can help ease tummy troubles and reduce inflammation.

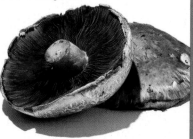

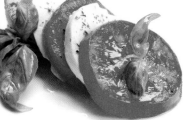

CAPRESE

A simple sandwich of mozzarella cheese and tomato will give you protein, heart-healthy lycopene, and almost half the calcium you need for your day.

CHEDDAR CHEESE WITH APPLE OR PEAR

The hearty crunch of fiber-rich fruit coupled with the calcium of the cheese make for a flavorful and super healthy lunch for you and your babe.

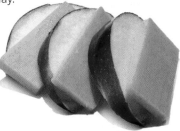

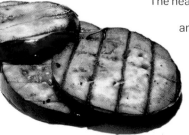

GRILLED EGGPLANT

The compounds that give eggplants their dark purple color help you fight off disease and also contribute to the healthy growth of your baby's brain cells. Oh, and did we mention they're low-fat and low-calorie?

Eat This
Panera Roasted Turkey Cranberry Flatbread,
served hot

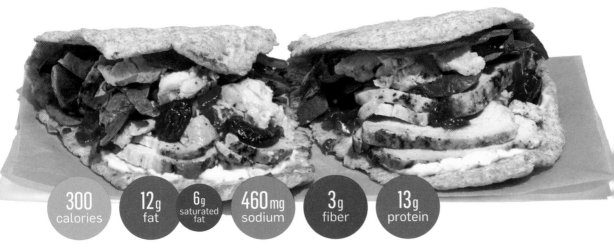

300 calories   **12g** fat   **6g** saturated fat   **460mg** sodium   **3g** fiber   **13g** protein

Not only does the schmear of cranberry sauce punch up the flavor profile of this sandwich, cranberries have also been known to help fight back against heartburn. And at just 300 calories, you'll still have room for dessert!

Good 'wiches

Quiznos
Turkey Lite on Artisan Wheat (Regular)
Cheers to the chain's "500 Calories or Less" menu— this sandwich included.

Au Bon Pain
Grilled Chicken Sandwich
Substantial, flavorful and packed with 32 grams of protein—yum.

Friendly's
Grilled Chicken Breast Burger
...with lettuce, tomato, and avocado. Build your own.

Scale Up on Flavor

Not That!
Panera Roasted Turkey, Apple, and Cheddar Sandwich

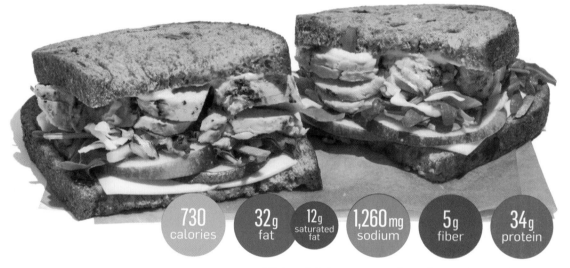

730 calories | **32g** fat | **12g** saturated fat | **1,260mg** sodium | **5g** fiber | **34g** protein

This pick has more than four times the amount of sodium as a large order of McDonald's fries. Aren't you feeling bloated enough as it is?

Wicked 'wiches

Quiznos Turkey Bacon Guacamole Sandwich (Large)
Normally, we'd say olé to guacamole, but this packs nearly two days' worth of salt.

Au Bon Pain Newport Turkey Sandwich
Sounds healthy—and would be, save for the cheddar and sugary honey mustard.

Friendly's Citrus Grilled Chicken Sandwich
Compared to the option on the left, this has twice the calories, twice the sodium, and four times the fat!

RULE #2:
Watch Out for the Health Halo

"Vegetarian" doesn't automatically translate to "healthy." Some sammies are packed with four different kinds of cheese, a deluge of oil, and sodium-packed veggie patties, stuffed inside a hulking 12" roll, resulting in a half a day's worth of calories and a cascade of carbs. Limit yourself to one or two types of cheese, endless undressed veggies, and a small bun.

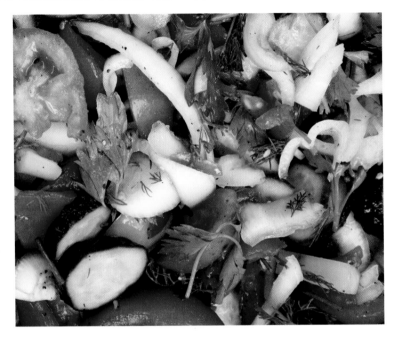

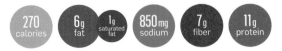

Eat This
Blimpie Veggie & Cheese Sub

Lettuce, tomato, onion, banana peppers, roasted red peppers, and black olives don't just give this sandwich a satisfying crunch, they also deliver a ton of amazing nutrients for you and baby—like vitamin C and lycopene.

270 calories	6g fat	1g saturated fat	850mg sodium	7g fiber	11g protein

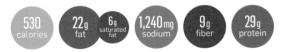

Not That!
Blimpie VegiMax

The veggie patty on this sandwich is laden with salt, and the creamy Italian dressing it's doused in doesn't help much, either. When it comes to veggies, you're almost always better off going for fresh ones.

530 calories	22g fat	6g saturated fat	1,240mg sodium	9g fiber	29g protein

RULE #3:
Don't Load Up on Extra Meat

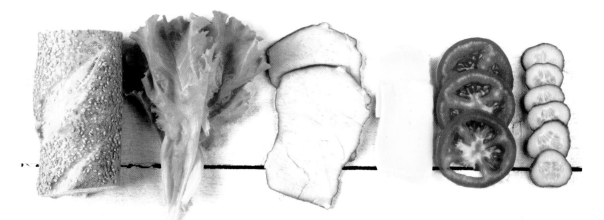

I've told you how important protein is to your baby's health. But I've also warned you about sodium. Piling on more than three slices of certain deli meats can add up to half a day's worth of salt. Limit the meat to less, and ask for low-sodium. Better yet: go for cooked tuna.

Eat This
Subway 6" Turkey Breast on 9-grain Wheat with Natural Cheddar Cheese, Lettuce, Tomato, and Mustard—served hot

Turkey isn't just a low-fat protein source, it also contains tryptophan, which can help squash sugar cravings and boost your mood.

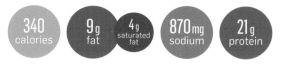

| 340 calories | 9g fat | 4g saturated fat | 870mg sodium | 21g protein |

Not That!
Subway Turkey Italiano Melt

Gobbling turkey during pregnancy is a great idea, but add salami and pepperoni to the mix and you've got an unhealthy meaty mess.

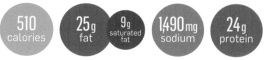

| 510 calories | 25g fat | 9g saturated fat | 1,490mg sodium | 24g protein |

THE SANDWICH MATRIX
Just remember to cook your deli meat!

Warning, each roll could pack up to 250 calories. Look for small, lighter, less-dense rolls. And don't be afraid to scoop out some of the excess bread.

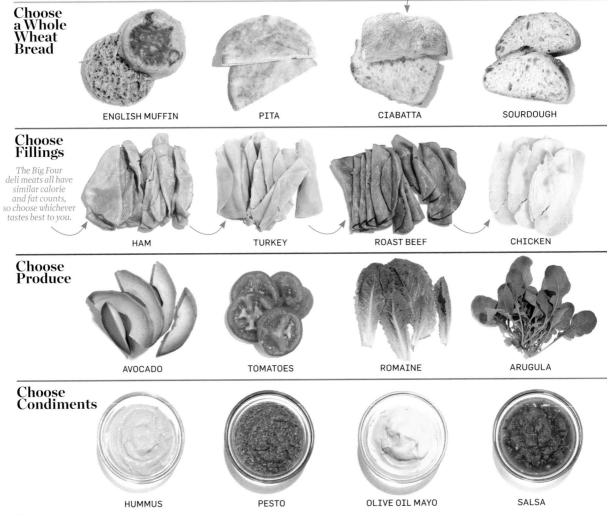

Choose a Whole Wheat Bread

ENGLISH MUFFIN   PITA   CIABATTA   SOURDOUGH

Choose Fillings

The Big Four deli meats all have similar calorie and fat counts, so choose whichever tastes best to you.

HAM   TURKEY   ROAST BEEF   CHICKEN

Choose Produce

AVOCADO   TOMATOES   ROMAINE   ARUGULA

Choose Condiments

HUMMUS   PESTO   OLIVE OIL MAYO   SALSA

*Rotisserie chicken is
perfectly suitable for
cold sandwiches,
but for a superlative
hot sandwich,
go with a freshly
grilled chicken breast
or thigh.*

*Pepperidge Farm makes the best of
the new wave of skinny sandwich breads.
At 100 calories and 5 grams of fiber,
their Deli Flats are at the top of the heap.*

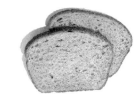

SANDWICH THINS

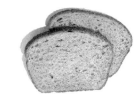

WHOLE-GRAIN BREAD

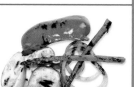

GRILLED CHICKEN

GRILLED VEGETABLES

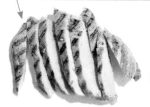

ROASTED RED PEPPERS

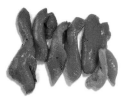

SLICED ONION

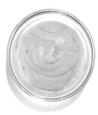

DIJON

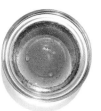

OIL AND VINEGAR

SUPER SANDWICHES

Choose the right bread and the right condiments
and a tasty 350-calorie sandwich is well within reach.
Make sure your next sandwich stacks up.

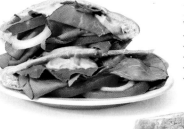

Power-up Pita
Whole-grain pita
+ hummus
+ roast beef
+ romaine
+ onion
+ tomato

BLTE
Toasted sourdough
+ arugula
+ tomato
+ nitrate-free bacon
+ sunny-side-up egg

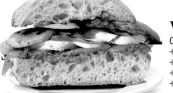

Vegapalooza
Ciabatta
+ grilled vegetables
+ roasted peppers
+ pesto-mayo
+ fresh mozzarella

Mexi Melt
English muffin
+ grilled chicken or turkey
+ Jack cheese
+ avocado
+ salsa

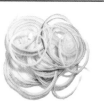

You're Craving Pasta

There's a good chance you spent your life before pregnancy limiting your carb intake, while watching your figure—but now, you'd kill for some Chef Boyardee. Find a happy medium. Pasta can be the perfect vehicle for baby-friendly veggies, fiber, and healthy fats, if done right.

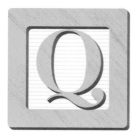

Q

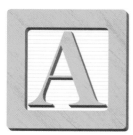

A

CAN I REALLY EAT PASTA?

Yes! Just always order whole wheat. Whole wheat pasta boasts mood-boosting B-vitamins and plenty of healthy fiber. Major bonus? It contains a compound called alpha-linolenic acid, which converts to omega-3 fatty acids in your body—and as I've said, those are majorly important in the development of your baby's brain. See, carbs are good for you—and her.

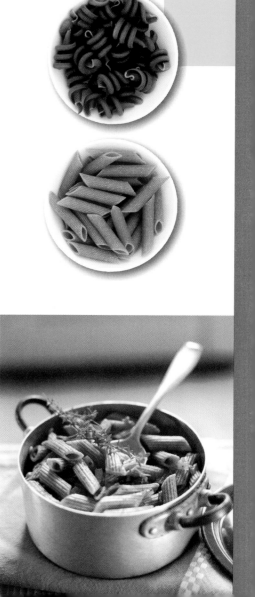

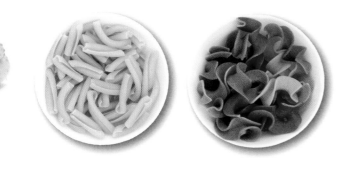

FEELING SAUCY
Which one is best for baby?

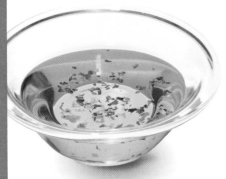

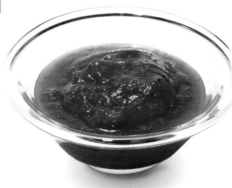

ALFREDO
What makes this stuff so delicious? Butter, heavy cream, and cheese. Sure, that means this white, creamy sauce has a decent amount of calcium, but with so much fat and an astronomical calorie count, you'd be better off getting that nutrient elsewhere!

OLIVE OIL
The simple, savory oil is full of healthy fats that can help baby's brain development and that will make your hair look its shiniest and most luxurious.

PESTO
Basil, one of the main ingredients in this green sauce, is a great source of choline, a nutrient that can protect baby's brain and boost your own brain power during pregnancy.

MARINARA
All those tomatoes in your favorite red sauce give you a great vitamin C blast, which will help baby's bones and teeth grow strong.

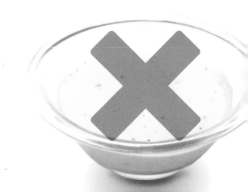

WIN THE BREAD BATTLE

Let's face it, your favorite Italian restaurant's ubiquitous bread bowl can be almost impossible to resist—but adding even more carbs to your meal can lead your sugar levels to spike, which isn't good for you or baby! Here's how to deal.

Ask your server to take the breadsticks away if you can—just make sure no one else at your table objects!

Order a side salad as an appetizer. That way, you'll have something fresh to nibble on while others are nomming on the bread.

Break bread—literally! Grab that roll you've got your eye on, ear it in half, and leave the rest in the basket. Easy peasy!

155

RULE #1: Eat Less by

![down arrow icon] **Eat This**

Olive Garden Cucina Mia! Spaghetti
with a half-serving of Primavera sauce

TWIRL THIS!

Olive Garden Create-Your-Own Pasta Bowl
Pair the whole wheat linguine with the marinara and grilled chicken—boom, guilt-free pasta.

Romano's Macaroni Grill Create Your Own Pasta
Here, you'll want the whole-wheat fettuccine, a touch of olive oil, asparagus and a roasted chicken.

Buca di Beppo Chicken Limone
It's on the gluten free menu. Just ask for the lemon butter sauce on the side.

635 calories   **25.5g** fat   **4g** saturated fat   **835mg** sodium

Add some vegetables to your pasta dish! Those who consume main dishes that incorporate veggies consume 350 fewer calories daily than those who eat their produce as a side dish, according to Penn State researchers. This meal has far too much sodium, but the veggies boost the amount of satiating fiber on your plate while also adding bulk.

Eating More

Not That!
Olive Garden Five Cheese Ziti al Forno

MAMMA MIA!

Olive Garden Eggplant Parmigiana
The eggplant's healthy. The oil it's fried in, not so much.

Romano's Macaroni Grill Mama's Trio
Not the mama! This is a cheesy, carby mess.

Buca di Beppo Chicken Carbonara
Prosciutto *and* Alfredo sauce? Celebrate with a bowl post-baby.

1,220 calories

71g fat

36g saturated fat

2,160mg sodium

While it's true that your body needs more fat during pregnancy than it did before you were expecting, nobody needs 71 grams of fat in one sitting! Yikes.

RULE #2:
Watch for Heavy Sauces

…you know, like the kind in fettuccine Alfredo. The Cheesecake Factory's chicken-filled take on the dish carries 2,300 calories and 103 grams of saturated fat. That's the fat equivalent of 51 Chicken McNuggets! Instead, get a marinara, and at home, make a creamy sauce by combining avocados, basil, garlic, olive oil, salt, pepper, and lemon juice in a food processor. You'll get healthy fats that can help lower cholesterol.

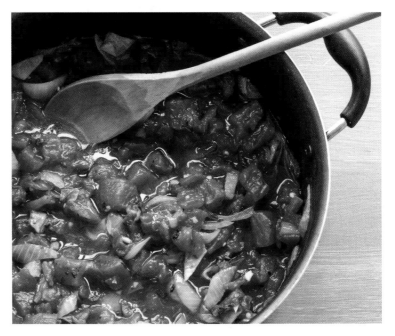

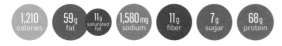

Eat This
California Pizza Kitchen
Asparagus and Spinach Spaghettini
with Grilled Chicken Breast

Only eat half of this, because of that insane sodium count, but overall, this isn't a bad choice—especially since the folate in asparagus can help prevent birth defects!

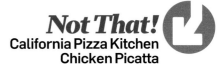

| 1,210 calories | 59g fat | 11g saturated fat | 1,580mg sodium | 11g fiber | 7g sugar | 68g protein |

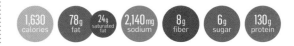

Not That!
California Pizza Kitchen
Chicken Picatta

Where'd all that fat come from? Look no farther than the sauce smothering the chicken in this way-too-indulgent dish.

| 1,630 calories | 78g fat | 24g saturated fat | 2,140mg sodium | 8g fiber | 6g sugar | 130g protein |

RULE #3:
Feeling Down? Lighten Up!

We all love hearty toppers like meat sauce, but some contain a shocking amount of sodium and fat. Spaghetti carbonara, for example, typically calls for thick-cut bacon, which carries about 70 calories and 6 grams of fat in two slices. If meat sauce is your go-to, cut calories and fat without changing the taste with two simple steps: Ask for ground chicken instead, and keep the sauce light.

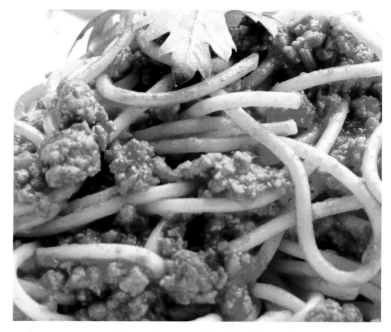

Eat This
T.G.I. Friday's Bruschetta Chicken Pasta

Twirl this pasta to your heart's content. Filled with fresh tomatoes and lean chicken, it'll leave you feeling light and energized!

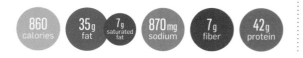

| 860 calories | 35g fat | 7g saturated fat | 870mg sodium | 7g fiber | 42g protein |

Not That!
T.G.I. Friday's Cajun Shrimp & Chicken Pasta

Shrimp and chicken are both great for you, but that heavy Alfredo-esque sauce kind of ruins the moment.

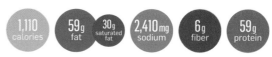

| 1,110 calories | 59g fat | 30g saturated fat | 2,410mg sodium | 6g fiber | 59g protein |

THE PASTA MATRIX
Go carb crazy—just pick the whole wheat.

They'll float to the top of the pot when they're done cooking.

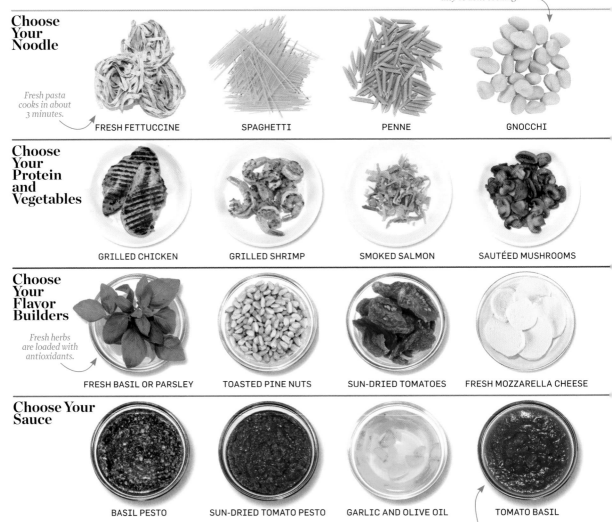

Choose Your Noodle

Fresh pasta cooks in about 3 minutes.

FRESH FETTUCCINE   SPAGHETTI   PENNE   GNOCCHI

Choose Your Protein and Vegetables

GRILLED CHICKEN   GRILLED SHRIMP   SMOKED SALMON   SAUTÉED MUSHROOMS

Choose Your Flavor Builders

Fresh herbs are loaded with antioxidants.

FRESH BASIL OR PARSLEY   TOASTED PINE NUTS   SUN-DRIED TOMATOES   FRESH MOZZARELLA CHEESE

Choose Your Sauce

BASIL PESTO   SUN-DRIED TOMATO PESTO   GARLIC AND OLIVE OIL   TOMATO BASIL

Muir Glen's Tomato Basil is one of the best sauces in the supermarket.

Other great vegetable add-ins include roasted asparagus, sautéed zucchini, caramelized onions, and diced eggplant.

Again, when possible, opt for whole wheat.

RIGATONI

FARFALLE

CHERRY TOMATOES

SAUTÉED SPINACH

RED PEPPER FLAKES

CHOPPED OLIVES

Why not add a pinch of metabolism-spiking dried chiles?

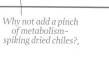

RED PEPPER ALFREDO

This rosy-hued cream sauce from Classico is the only acceptable jarred Alfredo sauce we've ever seen.

STANDBY PA

In the time it takes you to boil water an
you can whip up a sauce loaded with le
fresh vegetables, and antioxidant-dens
ers. Here are four favorites.

Yo

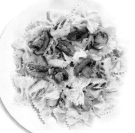

Pasta Milano
farfalle
+ grilled chicken
+ sautéed mushrooms
+ sun-dried tomatoes
+ toasted pine nuts
+ red pepper Alfredo

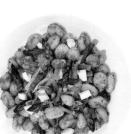
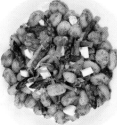

Gnocchi Romano
gnocchi
+ smoked salmon
+ asparagus
+ mozzarella
+ sun-dried tomato pesto

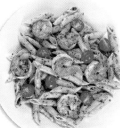

Penne Genovese
penne
+ grilled shrimp
+ cherry tomatoes
+ basil pesto

Sicilian Spaghetti
spaghetti
+ cherry tomatoes
+ pine nuts
+ olive oil & garlic
+ red pepper flakes
+ fresh basil

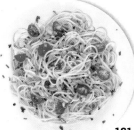

161

...u're Craving A Pizza

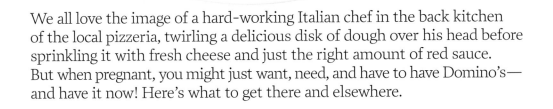

We all love the image of a hard-working Italian chef in the back kitchen of the local pizzeria, twirling a delicious disk of dough over his head before sprinkling it with fresh cheese and just the right amount of red sauce. But when pregnant, you might just want, need, and have to have Domino's— and have it now! Here's what to get there and elsewhere.

THE THIN AND THICK OF IT

Every healthy pizza starts with a healthy crust choice. Of course we all have our favorites, but knowing what's what will help you make smarter decisions for you and baby.

STUFFED CRUST

Hooboy. Watch out for this one—stuffed crust usually means its stuffed with extra fat and calories that can leave you feeling sluggish and gross.

NEW YORK STYLE

The thinner crust won't weigh you down, and will really let the toppings be the star of the show.

DEEP DISH

As a once in a while treat? Fine. As your go-to pie? Probably not, especially if you're dealing with gestational diabetes. Thick crusts mean you're eating a lot more bread, which can elevate your sugar levels.

WHOLE WHEAT

Just like whole wheat pasta or bread, whole wheat pizza crust has more fiber than the regular kind, which can keep you from feeling like you've got a brick in your belly in addition to baby!

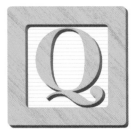

SO CAN I HAVE TWO SLICES?

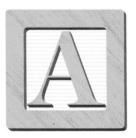

In other words, how much is too much of a good thing? Two to three slices, depending on your topping choices, can be totally fine for a big lunch or reasonable dinner, but watch out for those "personal sized" pizzas! They typically have about double the pizza that you should have in one sitting, so share with a friend or take some home for later.

Pepperoni Patrol

It might be the most popular topping in all of pizza history, but recent studies have shown cured meats like pepperoni to increase your risk of cancer. If you find one called "uncured" or "nitrate-free," it's good to go.

SURPRISING TOPPINGS TO ORDER TONIGHT

Don't hold back when ordering these amazing pie toppers!

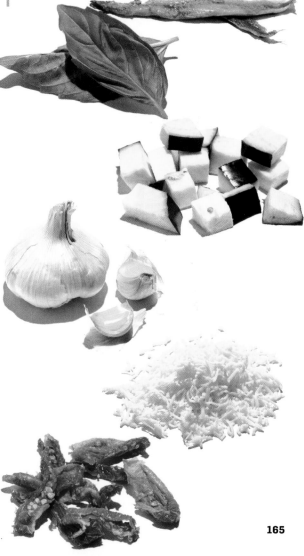

ANCHOVIES

These salty little guys are packed with brain-boosting omega-3 fatty acids and have even been said to help combat morning sickness.

BASIL

The iron in these green leaves can boost your energy so you can make it through that prenatal yoga class, no sweat!

EGGPLANT

These purple, meaty slices are super filling, low in calories, and high in fiber. A winning combination!

GARLIC

Getting a cold or the flu during pregnancy is the opposite of cute, so load up on immunity-boosting garlic to stay healthy and happy!

CHEESE

Enjoy all that melty goodness! Cheese is an excellent source of calcium, which is vital in pregnancy as it not only serves as the building blocks of baby's bone structure, but can also reduce your risk of preeclampsia by almost 50 percent.

SUNDRIED TOMATOES

These little beauties add a great texture to any pie, but they also pack a protein punch (who knew?!) that can help reduce muscle aches and pains.

RULE #1: Not all Veggie

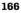 **Eat This**

Two slices of Pizza Hut Skinny Beach Pizza

400 calories

12g fat

6g saturated fat

860mg sodium

4g fiber

4g sugar

20g protein

Baby will love you for all the
healthy basil on this pizza,
and you'll love the satisfying taste.

☺ These Slices are Nice

**Sbarro New York Style
Fresh Tomato Pizza** (1 slice)
The bus station staple offers
this light and simple offering.

**Uno Chicago Grill Cheese
and Tomato Flatbread Pizza**
(½ pizza)
The key to (relative) success
at Uno's lies in their
flatbread pies—and share them!

CiCi's Cheese Flatbread
All the crunch,
less of the bread.

Pies Are Created Equal

560 calories

20 g fat

8 g saturated fat

1,280 mg sodium

4 g fiber

8 g sugars

24 g protein

Not That!
6-inch Pizza Hut Veggie Lover Personal Pan Pizza

The fat and sodium combo here will leave you feeling bloated and blah for the rest of the day.

These are Italia-nos

Sbarro Stuffed Sausage and Pepperoni Pizza (1 slice)
It's stuffed all right—with the fat equivalent of 10 slices of pan-fried bacon!

Uno Chicago Grill Chicago Classic Deep Dish Individual Pizza
The thick doughy base holds up extra heaps of cheese, sauce, and greasy toppings.

CiCi's Pizza Buffet Mac & Cheese
In CiCi's all-you-can-eat environment, the damage can add up quickly.

RULE #2:
Add More Veg, Not More Cheese

You can lower a pizza's Glycemic Index (GI)— a measure of how quickly blood glucose levels rise in response to a certain food—by adding fiber- and protein-rich toppings. For example, while a simple cheese pizza scores an 80 (out of 100), a veggie supreme pie clocks in at 49. Raw veggies and lean meats (chicken breast, ham) make for the best toppers.

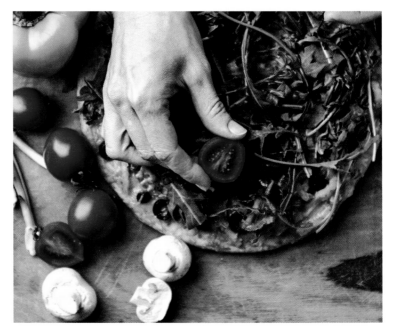

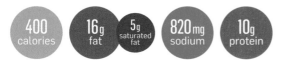

Eat This
Papa John's Mediterranean Veggie Thin Crust Pizza (2 slices of large)

With pizza this flavorful, you'll feel satisfied with just a couple slices— plus, onions are an anti-inflammatory food.

400 calories   **16g** fat   **5g** saturated fat   **820mg** sodium   **10g** protein

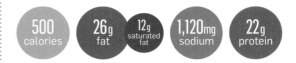

Not That!
Papa John's Tuscan Six Cheese Thin Crust Pizza (2 slices of large)

Cheese has a lot of calcium, which is great and all, but why miss an opportunity to get added nutrients?

500 calories   **26g** fat   **12g** saturated fat   **1,120mg** sodium   **22g** protein

RULE #3:
Go Thin—or Go Home!

Most of the evils of pizza lie in the empty-calorie, yet highly caloric crust. Typically made from refined white flour, pizza dough offers little nutrition to your body and will spike your insulin levels, causing you to crave more. The less crust you indulge in, the better. That means thin crust pizzas are almost always the better option.

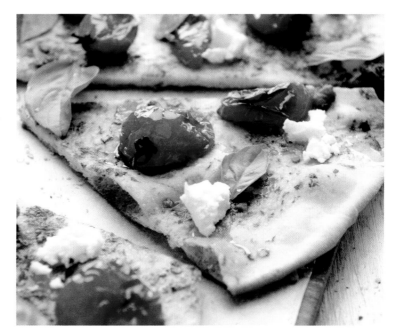

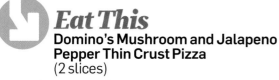

Eat This
Domino's Mushroom and Jalapeno Pepper Thin Crust Pizza
(2 slices)

Hey, hot mama! Those spicy peppers add a ton of flavor and can even help clear up a stuffy nose if you're not feeling so hot.

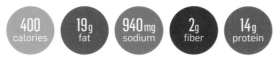

| 400 calories | 19g fat | 940mg sodium | 2g fiber | 14g protein |

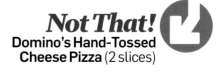

Not That!
Domino's Hand-Tossed Cheese Pizza (2 slices)

How did a zero-topping pizza lose out to one with yummy add-ons? You guessed it . . . the crust is the culprit!

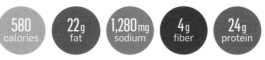

| 580 calories | 22g fat | 1,280mg sodium | 4g fiber | 24g protein |

You're Craving A Salad

People may claim that most cravings involve fatty, salty, not-good-for-you foods, but the truth of the matter is that sometimes your body just wants something that's simply fresh. A light, nutritious salad can make you feel healthier and more active from the very first crunch. Plus? It's an amazing way to get all the nutrients baby needs to grow strong and healthy. Toss that salad.

ALL ABOUT THAT BASE

You might think salads are all about what you put in them, but the greens you choose as your base are just as important. Here's how those leafy options measure up.

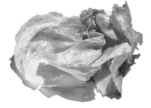

ICEBERG LETTUCE

If it's your only choice, know that it's not actually bad for you—but it's not doing you any favors, either.
This crunchy stuff is basically a bowl filled with blah: all water and no nutrients.

ROMAINE

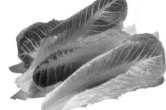

This leafier, softer green is a little better for you than its icy pal, so if you've only got the two options, go with this one.
It has a moderate amount of vitamin A, which, in measured amounts, is good for baby's development.

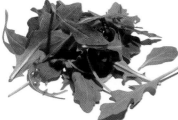

ARUGULA

This more flavorful leaf has a little more potassium than Romaine, which helps circulate all that extra blood you're carrying, and also boasts more fiber, protein, and vitamin C than Romaine. And? It has more bone-building calcium than any other leafy green.

SPINACH

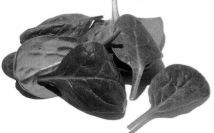

Popeye ate it for a reason! Spinach leaves have roughly 50 percent more potassium than Romaine, more fiber, and almost double the vitamin C. It's also the leader in iron levels among all leafy greens, so if you're anemic or are being told that you might need more iron, spinach might be your best bet.

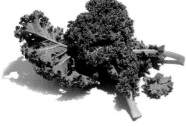

KALE

The rumors are true. Kale is, in fact, a superfood. How so? It's got over 50 percent more protein than any other salad base and roughly four times the vitamin C. Yes, it takes more chewing and a little getting used to, but once you go kale, you never go back!

SALAD DRESSING SHAKEDOWN

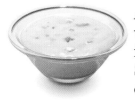

Almost all salad dressings will be safe for you and baby—with the exception, possibly, of restaurant-made Caesar dressing if it's made with raw eggs—but otherwise, you're A-OK. Still, not all of them are as healthy as others. Here's a quick rundown of what's what.

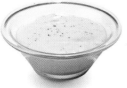

BLUE CHEESE

It's chunky, it's creamy, and it's . . . not surprisingly filled with a lot of fat and calories that neither you nor baby needs.

RANCH

This is another heavy hitter. If you've simply got to have your ranch, order it on the side and use sparingly, as it can contain all kinds of additives and artificial junk you don't want.

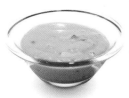

THOUSAND ISLAND

How would you feel about eating a giant tablespoon of mayo plus some ketchup right now? If you're not really okay with it, then rethink this choice, because that's just about what you're doing.

BALSAMIC VINAIGRETTE

This lighter option is relatively healthy compared to other choices. The olive oil in this contains plenty of healthy fats, and the vinegar adds a flavorful punch. Nice!

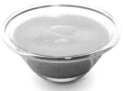

HONEY MUSTARD

This is a great choice, especially if it's restaurant made. Low in fat and calories, and high in flavor, you can't go wrong.

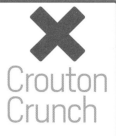

Crouton Crunch

Croutons might seem like an innocent added crunch on top of your salad, but the truth is, they're loaded with unhealthy fats and simple carbs that aren't good for you or baby. Opt for some sunflower seeds or even a few shaved almonds to top your salad instead!

TOSS THESE AROUND

Look for these power toppings at your local salad place to power up you and baby.

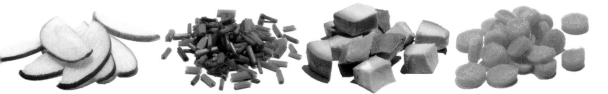

APPLES

You might not think of putting them in a salad, but they add a wonderful crunch and sweetness, and the fiber they give you can help keep you from feeling bloated and heavy.

CHIVES

These bad boys can help prevent painful leg cramps in pregnancy and will also boost your vitamin C and iron levels.

AVOCADO

The type of fat found in these tasty treats is incredibly important in developing your baby's healthy cells. Plus, they can help your skin stay pliable and stretchy as your bump grows.

CARROTS

They add a bit of color and crunch to your salad, and can help boost baby's vision as well as your own!

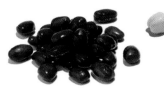

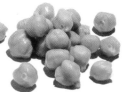

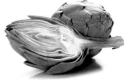

BLACK BEANS

These beans offer more than half of your daily needs in just one cup. Yes, please.

CHICKPEAS
or Garbanzo Beans

Did you know that in just one cup of these little guys, you get about a quarter of your daily protein and the same amount of your daily iron? Load them on!

ARTICHOKES

One medium artichoke hosts more than 10 percent of your daily folate needs. And since folate helps prevent birth defects, that's a biggie to watch for!

LENTILS

The protein in lentils can help keep your muscles strong and vital so you don't feel as worn down by the pregnancy weight.

RULE #1: Add Crunch

Eat This
Chili's Grilled Chicken Salad

Perfect for Salad Days

Applebee's Fiesta Chicken Chopped Salad
You don't need the dressing—the chicken comes glazed in chimichurri sauce.

McDonald's Premium Southwest Salad with Grilled Chicken
Hold the chili lime tortilla strips and it's even healthier.

Chili's Caribbean Salad with Grilled Chicken
The clean, lean chicken pairs nicely with the vitamin C-rich fresh pineapple.

430 calories

22g fat

6g saturated fat

1,090mg sodium

Light and delicious, the protein in this salad will keep you going even on your busiest day at work.

from the Garden ...not the fryer!

Put These on the Chopping Block

Applebee's Oriental Chicken Salad

Thanks to the sugary vinaigrette, crispy noodles and fried chicken, this has more calories, fat, and sugar than an order of Cheeseburger Eggrolls!

McDonald's Crispy Chicken Southwest Salad with Southwest Dressing

It's proudly made with real buttermilk and no artificial colors— but they never mention that it has 150 calories more than their grilled chicken breast.

Chili's Quesadilla Explosion Salad

This one's exploding— with trans-fats.

Not That!
Chili's Boneless Buffalo Chicken Salad

1,040 calories

72g fat

23g saturated fat

1,040mg sodium

Be cautious of any food that sounds unhealthy—with the word "salad" affixed at the end.

RULE #2: Half Portions Aren't Always Healthy

Why? Because half of something gross is still 100% gross. Check out the calorie, fat, and sodium count of the California Pizza Kitchen Moroccan-spiced salad below. (We're pretty sure Morocco would be annoyed to learn their top spice, according to CPK, is sugar.) To truly save calories, don't think about half-sizes or full; think first about the ingredients.

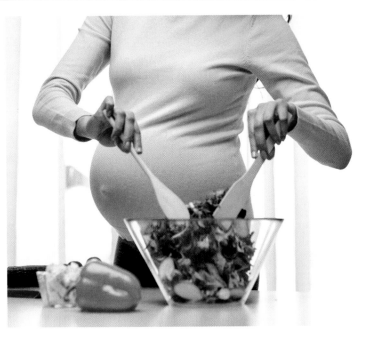

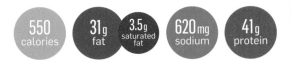

Eat This

California Pizza Kitchen Roast Veggie and Grilled Chicken Salad (Half portion)

Ask for the dressing on the side, and only use a few spoonfuls to keep calories and fat under lock.

550 calories	31g fat	3.5g saturated fat	620mg sodium	41g protein

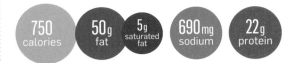

Not That!

California Pizza Kitchen Moroccan-Spiced Chicken Salad (Half portion)

Even just having a half-sized order is roughly the calories of a Big Mac and small fries.

750 calories	50g fat	5g saturated fat	690mg sodium	22g protein

RULE #3:
Keep It Clean!

If you're not a big lettuce fan, the only words worse than "I'll have a salad" may be "hold the dressing." But while some dressings are perfectly fine to eat—as I said on a previous page—even a honey mustard may have more than 200 hidden calories, since restaurants often blend theirs with high-fructose corn syrup. If trying to stay lean, make yours clean. Add yogurt instead.

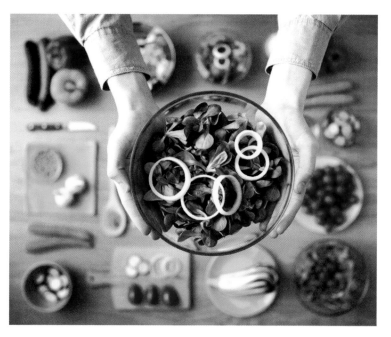

Eat This
Souplantation & Sweet Tomatoes
BBQ Julienne Chopped Salad (2 cups)
with Chicken and House-Made Fat-Free Ranch

This salad has plenty of flavor and protein to keep you satisfied, but has about a third of the fat of some options.

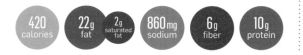

| 420 calories | 22g fat | 2g saturated fat | 860mg sodium | 6g fiber | 10g protein |

Not That!
Souplantation & Sweet Tomatoes
BBQ Smokehouse Salad (2 cups)
with Bacon and Peanuts

The added fat and sky-high sodium make this a no-no. Toss in bacon and it's even worse.

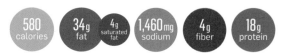

| 580 calories | 34g fat | 4g saturated fat | 1,460mg sodium | 4g fiber | 18g protein |

THE SALAD MATRIX
Mix and match your protein, fiber, and healthy fats.

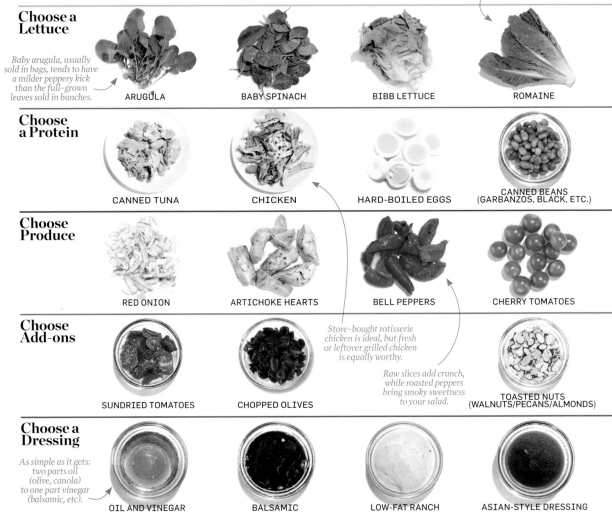

One of the most nutrient-packed lettuces available, teeming with vitamins K, A, and C

Choose a Lettuce

Baby arugula, usually sold in bags, tends to have a milder peppery kick than the full-grown leaves sold in bunches.

ARUGULA

BABY SPINACH

BIBB LETTUCE

ROMAINE

Choose a Protein

CANNED TUNA

CHICKEN

HARD-BOILED EGGS

CANNED BEANS
(GARBANZOS, BLACK, ETC.)

Choose Produce

RED ONION

ARTICHOKE HEARTS

BELL PEPPERS

CHERRY TOMATOES

Choose Add-ons

Store-bought rotisserie chicken is ideal, but fresh or leftover grilled chicken is equally worthy.

Raw slices add crunch, while roasted peppers bring smoky sweetness to your salad.

SUNDRIED TOMATOES

CHOPPED OLIVES

TOASTED NUTS
(WALNUTS/PECANS/ALMONDS)

Choose a Dressing

As simple as it gets: two parts oil (olive, canola) to one part vinegar (balsamic, etc.).

OIL AND VINEGAR

BALSAMIC

LOW-FAT RANCH

ASIAN-STYLE DRESSING

Turkey, ham, and roast beef are all welcome to the party—but cook them first.

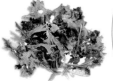

MIXED GREENS

ICEBERG

GRILLED STEAK

DELI MEAT

APPLE OR PEAR SLICES

AVOCADO

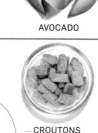

GRATED PARMESAN
(OR OTHER CHEESES)

CROUTONS

Whatever cheese you enjoy on your salad, make sure it is pasteurized.

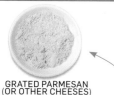

YOGURT

Yogurt dressing has a tang and creaminess that echoes ranch and blue cheese, without all the calories.

SUPER SALADS

Remember, you can never have too much produce in a salad.

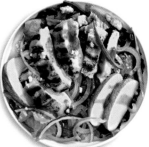

Apple-Blue
Bibb lettuce
+sliced red onion
+apple slices
+blue cheese
+chicken
+yogurt dressing

Mediterranean
Arugula
+tuna
+hard-boiled egg
+artichoke hearts
+roasted peppers
+chopped olives
+balsamic

Asian
Mixed greens
+cucumber
+mandarin oranges
+chicken
+chopped almonds
+ginger-soy dressing

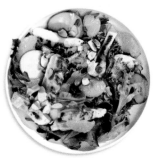

Chopped Salad
Shredded iceberg
+hard-boiled egg
+chopped ham
+cherry tomatoes
+shredded carrot
+red onion
+ranch

179

You're Craving Seafood

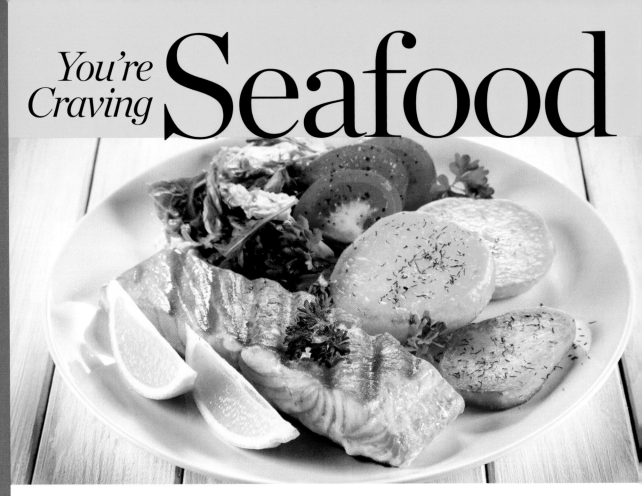

Whether it's the dead of winter or summer's in full swing, there's something about seafood that can take you right back to the breeziest of beach holidays—a feeling many of us could stand to remember while we're in the middle of pregnancy! And while you may have heard that fish are dangerous during pregnancy, most varieties are actually just fine. Here's how to know what's what and order safely the next time you've just gotta have a little surf with your turf!

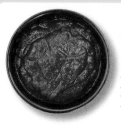

THE BIG DIPPERS

Fish like to swim . . . in yummy sauces!
Here's how to pick the best and leave the rest.

COCKTAIL SAUCE

is typically made of tomato paste, vinegar, and a number of spices. It's usually not too high in calories, but watch out for the sugars in this one, especially if you're eating one that came out of a bottle. Many of those are packed with high-fructose corn syrup, which isn't exactly great for you or baby!

TARTAR SAUCE

might add a creamy kick to your fish sticks, but it's anything but good for you. The premade stuff sometimes contains both corn syrup and high-fructose corn syrup,

and a hefty serving of vegetable oil. Additionally, it could contain raw egg, which could make you sick and lead to complications, so make sure to ask at restaurants before digging in.

MALT VINEGAR

is pretty much just what you think—aged vinegar! Because it doesn't have a lot of additives and junk in it, it's one of the better choices to dunk your fish in. Just be sure you don't let those fish go swimming in the stuff. A little is fine, but if you splash on more than a teaspoon or so, the sodium levels could make you feel puffy and bloated later on.

LEMON JUICE

is by far the healthiest addition to any seafood meal. It's all-natural, super flavorful, and adds a nice kick of vitamin C to your dinner. Plus, some women say lemon helps fight nausea. Nice!

THE ONLY FISH YOU NEED TO SKIP

Believe it or not, most fish are not dangerous for you during pregnancy. But avoid the below, which are high in mercury, and can cause major problems in your baby's development, including brain damage and hearing and vision problems.

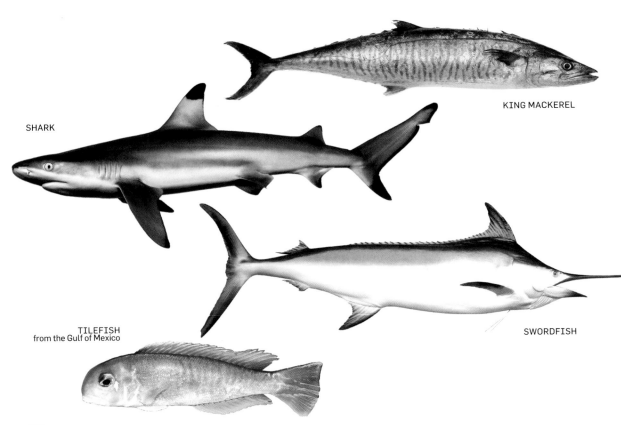

KING MACKEREL

SHARK

TILEFISH
from the Gulf of Mexico

SWORDFISH

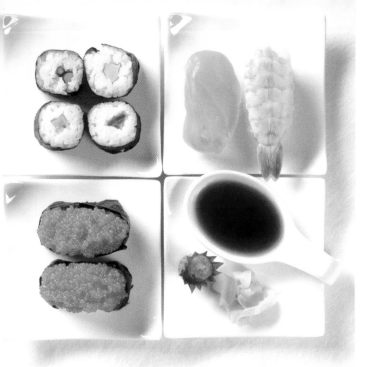

THE TRUTH ABOUT SUSHI

There's a lot of conflicting information out there. What's true? What's not?

A glass of wine every night, a nicely grilled swordfish steak, deli meat straight from the package, uncooked—of all the foods and drinks you shouldn't eat or drink during pregnancy, I missed sushi the most. But unfortunately you, too, have to say no-no to nori. No exceptions, no cheating.

Why? Because there's a chance that raw fish could contain parasites or bacteria that could lead to harmful infections. It's true that women in Japan and other countries continue to eat raw fish throughout their pregnancies, and routinely give birth to healthy babies, but as I tell my patients, why take the chance?

RULE #1: Salads Can Be

Eat This

Red Lobster Wood Grilled Fresh Salmon
Unsalted Baked Potato with Sour Cream, and a Side of Broccoli

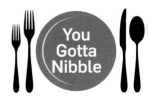

You Gotta Nibble

Chili's Ancho Salmon
From the "lighter choice" menu, this is one swimmingly good salmon.

Applebee's Savory Cedar Salmon
It's just 530 calories. But ask for the artichoke and lemon spread on the side.

Denny's Alaska Salmon
Simple. And better for you than their all-day pancakes.

585 calories

23g fat

5.5g saturated fat

465mg sodium

40g protein

When you get nice lean salmon on its own, you've still got plenty of room for potatoes, broccoli and even some sour cream.

Sneaky

Something's Fishy Here

Chili's Mango-Chile Tilapia
Although not an official no-no during pregnancy, tilapia is farmed under conditions that make them high in heart-unhealthy omega-6 fats. (You want omega-3s.)

Applebee's Double Crunch Shrimp
Twice-fried shrimp served with French fries?

Denny's Fish & Chips
The fish is fried. The chips are fried. This is gonna be delicious—after you have your baby.

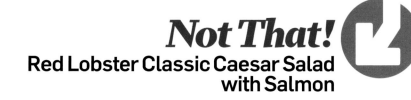

Not That!
Red Lobster Classic Caesar Salad with Salmon

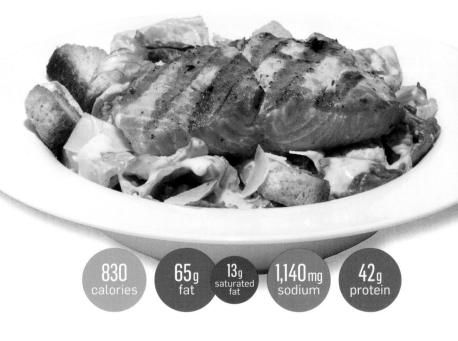

830 calories	65g fat	13g saturated fat	1,140mg sodium	42g protein

The dressing is what really kills this salad—and makes it have three times more fat than the choice with a yummy baked potato.

RULE #2:
Stay Cool on the Carbs

Obviously, if you want seafood, enjoy seafood—without the bread or fries. And don't be tempted by shrimp tempura: Its exotic countenance conceals that it's essentially french-fried sushi, or fish-and-chips without the chips. Meanwhile, the vegetable tempura at the Ra Sushi chain has an eye-popping 1,500 calories and 103 grams of fat.

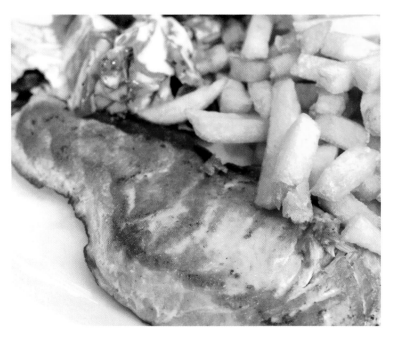

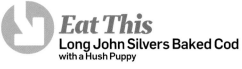

Eat This
Long John Silvers Baked Cod
with a Hush Puppy

The chips shouldn't be an everyday choice, but once in a while, they're a totally fine way to indulge.

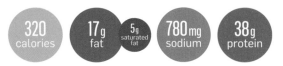

320 calories	17g fat	5g saturated fat	780mg sodium	38g protein

Not That!
Long John Silvers
Ciabatta Jack Fish Sandwich

Almost a hundred extra calories with a fraction of the protein and nearly triple the fat? You can blame the large serving of bread and dressings for all of that.

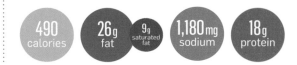

490 calories	26g fat	9g saturated fat	1,180mg sodium	18g protein

RULE #3:
Go Grilled Whenever You Can

The cardinal rule when eating out is that if it's not a simple grilled fillet, skip it. Applebee's New England Fish & Chips packs 1,970 calories and 136 grams of fat, while PF Chang's Kung Pao Scallops has 870 calories and 50 grams of fat. You'd be better off eating two McDonald's Filet-o-Fish. (Don't!) A twist of lemon and pepper is all you need to bring out the savory creaminess of salmon, or a nice grilled shrimp.

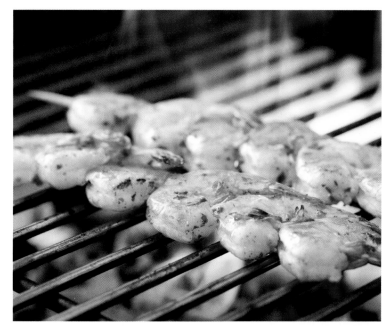

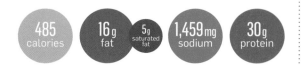

Eat This
Captain D's Seafood Kitchen Grilled Shrimp Skewers (2) with Cocktail Sauce, Corn on the Cob, and a Hush Puppy

Yes, you can have it all! This delicious and filling meal proves it.

Not That!
Captain D's Seafood Kitchen Southern Style White Fish Filet

Holy moly. No sides, no anything extra, and you've got more than three times the fat? Simply not worth it.

485 calories	16g fat	5g saturated fat	1,459mg sodium	30g protein

540 calories	37g fat	7g saturated fat	1,430mg sodium	26g protein

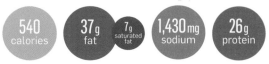

You're
Craving
Chicken

It's the ultimate down-home southern comfort food—and it's one of the healthiest proteins out there if you order smart. Here's how to get your chicken fix without flying the coop.

ORDER RIGHT, EVERY TIME

Fried chicken is okay as a once-in-a-while indulgence, but for every day, you'll want to be more strategic in your order. These three tips will help you keep things in order.

SKIP THE SKIN
Most of the fat in chicken is held in the skin. Ask for it skinless or just take the skin off once you get it to avoid a greasy, oily meal.

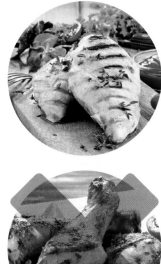

BREAST IS BEST
You've heard the saying in terms of breastfeeding, but it's true in terms of ordering your dinner as well! The breast meat in chicken is more muscular, which means it boasts more protein and less fat than other part.

GO LIGHT ON THE DRUMS
Drumsticks and thighs have a lot more fat on them than the breast. That doesn't mean you shouldn't eat them, but if those are your favorite parts, go for a smaller portion than you would otherwise.

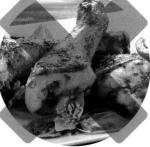

SMART SIDES
CHICKEN IS NOTHING WITHOUT A DELISH SIDE DISH OR TWO. HERE'S HOW TO MAKE THOSE EXTRA BITES COUNT.

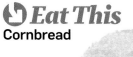 **Eat This**
Cornbread

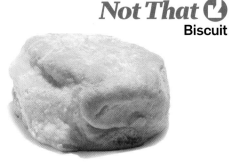 **Not That**
Biscuit

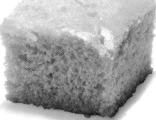

Neither one is actually that great for you, but at least the cornbread has more fiber, which can help prevent bloat and keep you feeling energized.

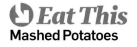 **Eat This**
Mashed Potatoes

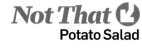 **Not That**
Potato Salad

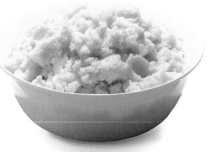

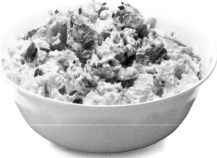

Potatoes are a great source of potassium, which is great for your (and baby's!) nerves and muscles. Just go easy on the fatty gravy, and try to skip the mayo-filled potato salad . . . who knows how long it's been sitting there, and besides, it's filled with unhealthy fats and additives.

Eat This
Steamed Broccoli

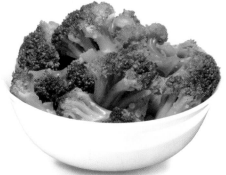

Not That
Creamed Corn

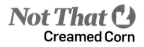

Creamed corn is yummy and not all that bad for you, but it's not that strong nutrient-wise. Meanwhile, steamed broccoli has protein, fiber, and a ton of vitamin C. Just another reason to eat your trees!

Eat This
Mac & Cheese

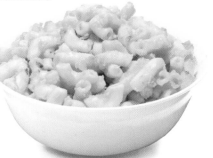

Not That
Cole Slaw

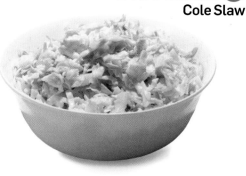

You might think the "salad" option would be healthier, but because the cole slaw is swimming in white dressing, it's a pretty close match to the cheesy pasta in terms of calories, and doesn't even have the calcium benefits that'll help baby's bones grow strong.

RULE #1: When Fried,

Eat This

Chick-Fil-A Chicken Sandwich

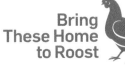

Bring These Home to Roost

McDonald's Artisan Grilled Chicken Sandwich
Remove the bun—and add a side salad and fresh mandarin orange—for the perfect meal.

Chipotle Chicken Bowl with Brown Rice
Chipotle's chickens are raised on a pasture (or in deeply-bedded pens) and are both antibiotic and hormone-free.

Applebee's Cedar Grilled Lemon Chicken
Come for the protein-packed chicken quinoa, stay for the sweet Granny Smith apple relish.

440 calories

18g fat

4g saturated fat

1,390mg sodium

The sodium level here is off the charts, but if you're really needing that deep-fried crunch, this is the way to go.

Pick the Sandwich

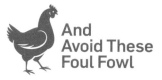

And Avoid These Foul Fowl

McDonald's Premium Buttermilk Crispy Chicken Deluxe Sandwich
At most fast food chains, "crispy" is code for "breaded with sugar and fried in fat."

Chipotle Chicken Soft Flour Tacos
When at Chipotle, do a chicken bowl, or even burrito—the soft tacos are too salty.

Applebee's Fiesta Lime Chicken
They should call it what it is: cheese nachos with a chicken breast crashing the party.

Not That!
Chick-Fil-A Cobb Salad
with Avocado Lime Ranch Dressing

500 calories

27 g fat

7 g saturated fat

1,360 mg sodium

Because there's more surface area, there's more fat and fried bread covering the chicken. You'd be better off with the sandwich.

RULE #2:
Pair Your Protein—Wisely

The best advice for pregnant moms eating out? Remembering what your mom told you, last time she served a chicken dinner. Eat your protein. (Chicken breast, preferably skinless—check.) Finish your vegetables. (Ideally steamed, not fried.) And enjoy a healthy starch. (Without too much butter.) Anything else— heavy sauces, crispy chips, onion straws, pot pies— and no dessert for you!

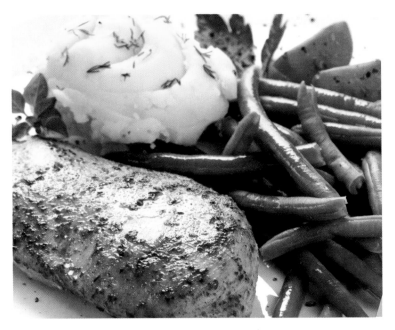

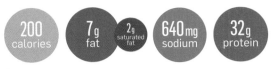

Eat This
KFC Kentucky Grilled Chicken Breast

It may not be the Colonel's original recipe but it's deliciously grilled.

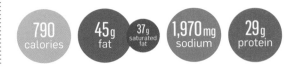

Not That!
KFC Chunky Chicken Pot Pie

This little pie packs over double the fat of a full meal with mashed potatoes and gravy? Something's really wrong here.

200 calories	7g fat	2g saturated fat	640mg sodium	32g protein

790 calories	45g fat	37g saturated fat	1,970mg sodium	29g protein

RULE #3:
Skip the 'Salad'

Salad's healthy. Chicken's healthy. So why is a chicken salad not cool? If you know how to make it, you already know the answer—it's traditionally full of mayo. One cup of chicken salad from Chick-Fil-A, for example, is coated in it, which is why it's got 24 grams of fat. In comparison, a whole Grilled Chicken Sandwich has just 5 grams.

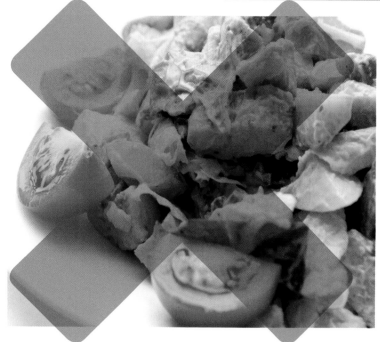

Eat This
One Quarter of a White Skinless Boston Market Rotisserie Chicken
with Cornbread and Green Beans

We'll gladly skip the skin in favor of some yummy cornbread.

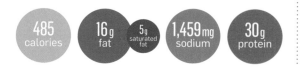

485 calories | 16g fat | 5g saturated fat | 1,459mg sodium | 30g protein

Not That!
Boston Market All White Chicken Salad Sandwich

Wait, all you get is a measly sandwich and it's got over 900 calories and almost five times the fat of the other meal? No thanks.

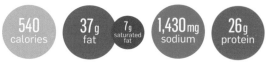

540 calories | 37g fat | 7g saturated fat | 1,430mg sodium | 26g protein

You're Craving Pan-Asian

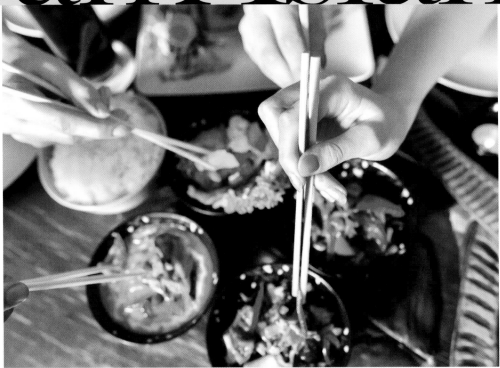

Traditional Chinese and Thai food is light and airy. But we don't live in China. In America, Pan-Asian cuisine can be loaded with salt—in fact, a mere tablespoon of traditional soy sauce has almost half a day's worth of sodium. Downing too much can lead to hypertension, a condition that restricts blood flow. Look for the "low sodium" option on your menus—and use this guide before picking up those chopsticks.

AGAINST THE GRAIN

Don't think what type of rice you choose matters that much? Think again.

STEAMED WHITE RICE

While one cup of this stuff serves up about 4 grams of protein, it's mainly just simple carbs—which, if you eat a lot of them, can lead to excess weight gain and the pregnancy complications that go along with that.

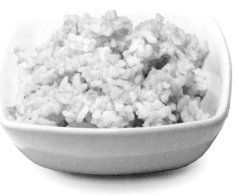

STEAMED BROWN RICE

While brown rice is also a carbohydrate, it's got a lot more going for it—including a hefty dose of fiber, a boost of protein, and even some blood-boosting iron. This is the best choice.

FRIED RICE

Full disclosure? Fried rice is delicious. Go ahead and have it once in a while if it's your favorite, but just know that you're not getting the nutrients you and baby need while chowing down on this stuff. Make up for it with plenty of colorful veggies later on.

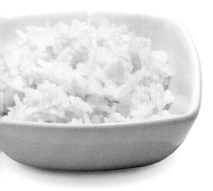

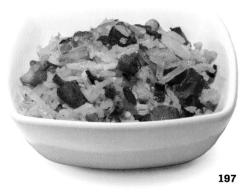

WHAT'S THE DEAL WITH MSG?

And will it hurt your baby?

MSG, properly known as mono-sodium glutamate, is a flavor additive often found in savory dishes at Chinese restaurants (and in many chips, like Pringles). The Food and Drug Administration has deemed it generally safe even for pregnant women, but I say avoid it if possible.

MSG increases appetite by blocking the message to the brain that you've eaten your fill. In fact, one group of researchers found that giving laboratory rats MSG increased their food intake by a whopping 40 percent! Worse, the chemical tells your body to pump out insulin, the fat-storage hormone. This surge of insulin causes your blood sugar to plummet and your hunger to return—with a vengeance. The great news is that a lot of restaurants have proudly ditched MSG. Look for notes on the menu.

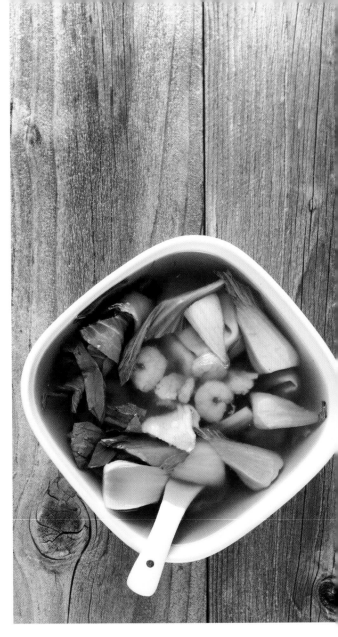

JUST SAY NO TO THESE NOMS

It's all yummy, we know that, but there are a few things baby wants you to skip at your fave Pan-Asian spot.

REGULAR SOY SAUCE

The salt levels here are insane! Go for the low-sodium kind instead. It tastes no different and won't send your blood pressure on a rollercoaster ride!

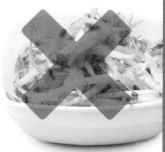

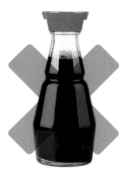

FRIED DUMPLINGS

Steamed dumplings are just as delish (if not even better) and they've got way fewer unhealthy fats.

EGG DROP SOUP

This might be a big sacrifice, but the egg here might not be fully cooked, which could put you and baby at risk of illness or bigger complications.

VEGETABLE TEMPURA

Yeah, there are technically veggies inside—but with that deep-fried coating, you may as well be eating a donut!

RAW BEAN SPROUTS

They seem healthy, but the truth is these might be harboring bacteria that could make you and your soon-to-be kiddo very sick. Make sure all bean sprouts are fully cooked before digging in!

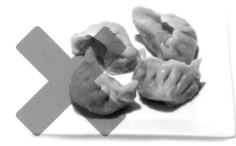

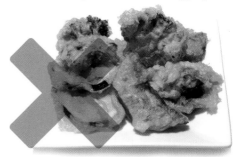

RULE #1: Go Easy on the

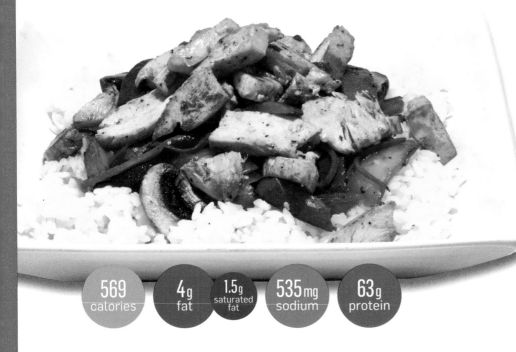

Eat This
Benihana Hibachi Lemon Chicken
with Shrimp Appetizer, Steamed Rice, and Zucchini

569 calories

4g fat

1.5g saturated fat

535mg sodium

63g protein

Surf and turf has never look healthier or more delicious, because the rice is steamed—instead of sauteed in oil, like the noodles on the right.

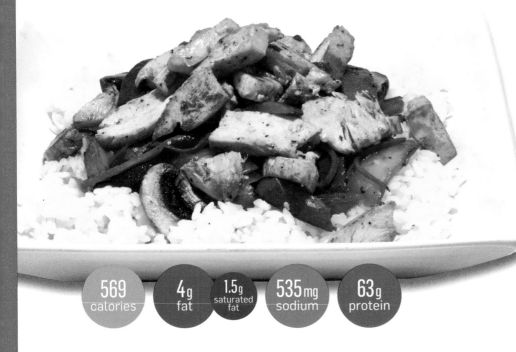

GOOD Chinese

Manchu Wok Pineapple Chicken
Enjoy the vitamin C and sweet kick of pineapple for only 170 calories.

Applebee's Thai Shrimp Salad
The chilis may be too spicy for your digestion, but this is a low-cal meal that satisfies.

Ruby Tuesday's Thai Phoon Shrimp
Ordered alone, these little guys aren't too bad—at only 205 calories.

Noodles

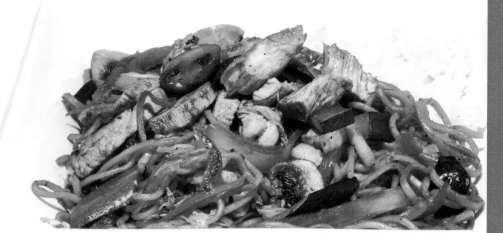

Not That! ↻
Benihana Chicken Yakisoba Dinner

BAD
Chinese

Manchu Wok Oriental Grilled Chicken
The calories are fine (at 240), but there's more sodium here than in 50 Ritz crackers!

Applebee's Shrimp Wonton Stir-Fry
Shrimp is great—when it's grilled. Here, it's fried in 1,630 mg of sodium.

Ruby Tuesday's International Shrimp Trio
Shrimp done three ways (including Thai style), two of them bad. This dish has 1,475 calories and 3,743 mg of sodium! That's more salt than 200 Doritos.

620 calories	10.5g fat	1g saturated fat	1,355mg sodium	36g protein

With high-protein, low-sodium options on Benihana's menu, why order the dish boiled in oil?

RULE #2:
Add Color to Your Plate

The more veggies, the better. "When faced with a takeout menu, I'd go for Buddha's Delight, with mounds of steamed vegetables and tofu for protein," says Marisa Moore, MBA, RDN, LD. "Chicken and broccoli is another good option; just be sure to keep your rice portion in check. And if you're dining in the restaurant, take advantage of the hot tea. It cleanses the palate and signals the brain that you're done eating."

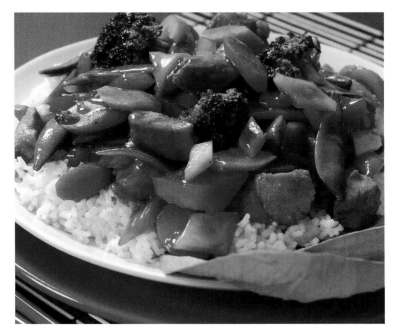

Eat This
Panda Express Kung Pao Chicken
Entree with Steamed Rice and Mixed Veggies

You're getting broccoli, carrots, zucchini, and a nice portion of protein—we think it can slide, as long as it's not an everyday meal, due to the sodium.

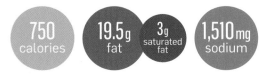

750 calories | 19.5g fat | 3g saturated fat | 1,510mg sodium

Not That!
Panda Express Orange Chicken
Entree with Chow Mein

When your plate looks as beige as this, it's going to be pretty blah nutritionally, too. Blame the fried noodles for the high fat content.

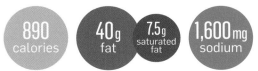

890 calories | 40g fat | 7.5g saturated fat | 1,600mg sodium

RULE #3:
Salty Sauces Are Not Superfoods

Even when she's not pregnant, "I always skip the sauce," says Lori Zanini, RD, CDE. "Chinese restaurants are notorious when it comes to adding excessive amounts of salt to their food. And I choose the safe foods. Most Chinese restaurants offer steamed vegetables and brown rice. I try to fill half the plate with the veggies and fill about ¼ the plate with brown rice. This will dramatically lower calories and fat of your dish."

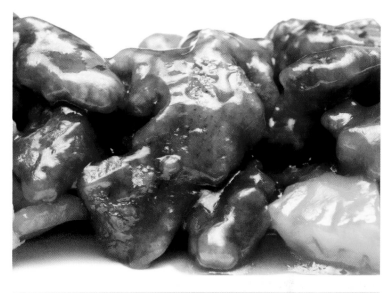

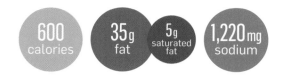

Eat This
PF Chang's Asian Grilled Salmon
with Grilled Asparagus and Red Pepper Slaw

Of all the seafood dishes at this chain, this one has the least amount of sodium.

600 calories	35g fat	5g saturated fat	1,220mg sodium

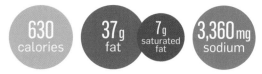

Not That!
PF Chang's Ooling Chilean Sea
Bass with Spinach

This dish has more salt than 20 servings of Lay's Potato Chips. Unless you want to feel even puffier and more swollen, step away from this dish!

630 calories	37g fat	7g saturated fat	3,360mg sodium

You're Craving
Ice Cream

Here is is. Here we are. The reason you bought the book. Ice cream and the eating of it. It's the number one craving among my patients (more than pickles, chips and even chocolate!). As I said in my introduction, yes, you can eat ice cream. It's loaded with calcium, can cool you off and, despite being high in fat and sugar, isn't unhealthy if eaten in moderation. Have a scoop in a cake cone. Just don't have three and top it with sprinkles, Swedish fish and five more scoops.

FOUR SUPER SHAKES

Milk shakes don't need to be 1,000-calorie calamities. Choose a base, complement it with one or two fillings, and add just enough liquid to bring it all together. Insert straw. Enjoy.

PBC
1 ripe frozen banana
+ ¾ cup low-fat milk
+ 1 cup chocolate frozen yogurt
+ ½ Tbsp peanut butter
+ 3 ice cubes

Strawberry Shortcake
1 cup strawberry ice cream
+ ½ cup frozen strawberries
+ ½ cup low-fat milk
+ 3 vanilla wafers
+ a bit of whipped cream on top

Raspberry Mango Madness
2 cups frozen mango
+ 1 cup raspberry sorbet or sherbet
+ ½ cup milk

Peaches and Cream
1 cup vanilla frozen yogurt
+ 1 cup frozen peaches
+ ½ cup milk

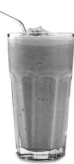

RULES OF THE MILK SHAKE

RULE 1
Build a better base.
Start with ice cream or frozen yogurt with less than 150 calories a scoop. Breyers Natural and Stonyfield Frozen Yogurt products are our favorite milk-shake makers.

RULE 2
Stretch it out.
Make ice cream the bulk of your milk shake and you're asking for trouble. Frozen fruit, juice, Greek yogurt, and ice all help you get more mileage out of your shake.

RULE 3
Sneak in nutrition.
Milk shakes don't need to be all ice cream, cookies, and candy. Frozen fruits add natural sweetness, they give the shake a rich, creamy body, and they can add a serving or two of much-needed produce to your drink.

RULE 4
Power up: A strong blender is essential.
A weak blender will only melt the ice cream (and ice, if using) and dilute your masterpiece. An Oster Classic Beehive Blender, sold for around $70, is perfect for all your milk shake and smoothie needs.

RULE #1: When You Order,

Eat This

Banana Peanut Butter Greek Frozen Yogurt
(½ cup)

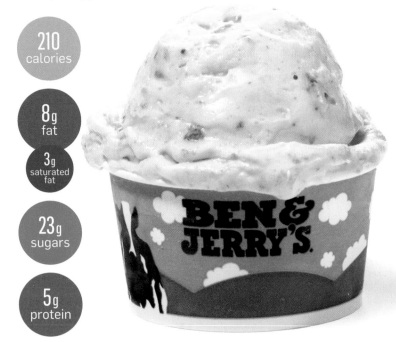

210
calories

8g
fat

3g
saturated
fat

23g
sugars

5g
protein

**We're
Getting
Chills**

**Baskin-Robbins
Soft Serve Cookie
Sandwich**
At just 180 calo-
ries, this is one
cookie puss we
wanna kiss.

**Cold Stone
Creamery Double
Chocolate Devo-
tion Cupcake**
You won't find
many "Eat This"
choices at this
chain, but here's
one indulgence we
can't resist.

**Dairy Queen Hot
Fudge Sundae
(small)**
Traditional sun-
daes are often the
most prudent
treats here.

Greek fro yo—newish to the menu—offers the same
creamy goodness of regular ice cream, minus most of the
saturated fat.

Go Greek

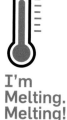

I'm Melting. Melting!

Baskin-Robbins Peanut Butter 'n Chocolate
This chain has a lighter menu, with frozen yogurt and no-sugar-added ice cream. Choose those, not this.

Cold Stone Creamery Brownie a La Cold Stone
...with as much fat as you'd find in a cup of mayo.

Dairy Queen Georgia Mud Fudge Blizzard (small)
Triple the fat and double the calories of a sundae.

Not That!
Peanut Butter Cup Ice Cream
(½ cup)

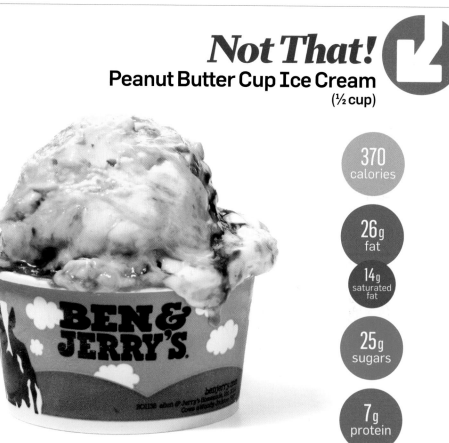

370 calories

26 g fat

14 g saturated fat

25 g sugars

7 g protein

Ben and/or Jerry managed to cram more than half a day's saturated fat into this peanut butter-chocolate bomb, making it the worst scoop on the menu.

SUNDAE MATRIX
Mmm...butter pecan.

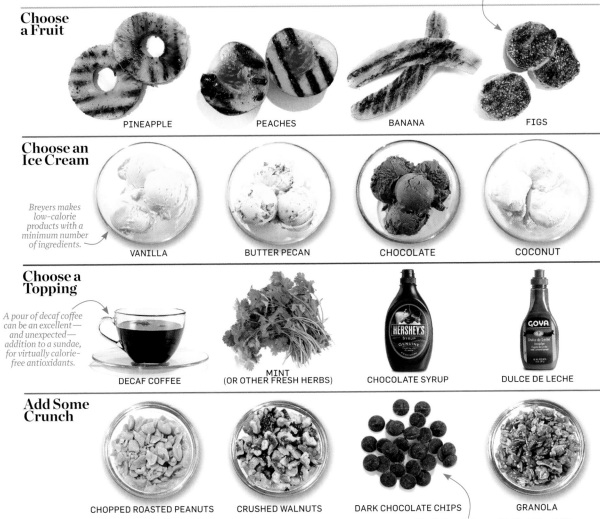

Other stone fruits like apricots and plums work just as well on the grill.

Choose a Fruit

PINEAPPLE PEACHES BANANA FIGS

Choose an Ice Cream

Breyers makes low-calorie products with a minimum number of ingredients.

VANILLA BUTTER PECAN CHOCOLATE COCONUT

Choose a Topping

A pour of decaf coffee can be an excellent— and unexpected— addition to a sundae, for virtually calorie-free antioxidants.

DECAF COFFEE MINT (OR OTHER FRESH HERBS) CHOCOLATE SYRUP DULCE DE LECHE

Add Some Crunch

CHOPPED ROASTED PEANUTS CRUSHED WALNUTS DARK CHOCOLATE CHIPS GRANOLA

The darker, the better. We like Ghirardelli's 60% Cacao Bittersweet Chocolate Baking Chips.

ONE SEC RECIPES

Mix and match fruit, ice cream, and add-ons however you like; there are literally hundreds of different paths to deliciousness. These four here just happen to be among our favorites.

Peaches and Cream

Grilled peaches
+ butter pecan ice cream
+ granola

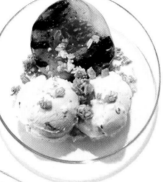

The Elvis

Banana
+ peanut butter ice cream
+ chocolate sauce
+ crushed peanuts

Piña Colada

Pineapple
+ coconut ice cream
+ dulce de leche
+ coconut flakes

ON THE BARBIE

The grill does magical things to fruit, softening its flesh, concentrating its natural sweetness, and transforming it into something that feels like dessert on its own. Trick it out with ice cream and a few toppings and you have a world-class sundae on your hands.

RULE 1

Grill fruit with the same attentiveness with which you grill steak. You don't want to blast the fruit so the heat melts it into mush. You want fruit that is caramelized and soft on the outside, but with a bit of bite in the center. For most fruit, that means 10 minutes tops on the grill.

RULE 2

The interplay of hot and cold is what makes this dessert so special. Have the ice cream at the table, slightly softened, ready to be scooped shortly after the fruit comes off the grill.

RULE 3

Use salty (roasted peanuts, granola) and bitter (green tea, a drizzle of olive oil) ingredients to cut through the sugar of the fruit and ice cream; it makes for a more interesting dessert.

RULE 4

Use small bowls and spoons. A study from Cornell University found that people who used both ate 30 percent less ice cream than people who used big bowls and spoons.

209

EAT THIS, NOT THAT! Special Report

SNEAKY SECRETS THE RESTAURANTS DON'T WANT YOU TO KNOW

If being an anonymous blip on a giant corporation's assembly line makes you feel like a character in some bleak sci-fi movie, I've got good news. There are plenty of ways to fight back—to enjoy all the convenience of modern restaurants and all the foods you still like to eat without harming your baby.

You see, all major restaurant chains—from the fast-food purveyors to the sandwich shops and coffee bars to the sit-down dinner joints with their vaguely Italian/Mexican/Chinese/whatever themes—operate with the same set of secrets, secrets they don't want their customers to know. And if you know these secrets, well, guess what? The power

to eat what you want and still stay slim is in your hands. Lucky you!

Here's how to start taking back control.

REMEMBER, THE WAITER IS A SALESPERSON

A 2005 study published in the Journal of Retailing and Consumer Services found that you're more likely to order a side dish when the server verbally prompts you. ("Do you want fries with that?") Restaurants know this, and now you know it, too. When the waiter makes a suggestion, remember his job is not to make you happy. His job is to extract money from your wallet and insert fat in its place.

DON'T GET TOO EXCITED

A 2008 study in the International Food Research Journal found that people are less likely to make healthy restaurant choices when they feel that they're dining out for a "special occasion." Before you head out to your next meal, really take stock of how many times you've eaten out this week. If you're eating every meal at home and dining out truly is a once-a-week splurge, then don't worry about it so much. But if you're like most of us, eating out is probably more like a once-a-day splurge. And if that's the case, remember, there's nothing special here. Eat smart today because you'll have to do it again tomorrow.

START SMALL

Here's the good news: No one is going to stop you from ordering seconds. So be like any good businessperson, and start small. Speaking of which:

DON'T GET "SUPERSIZED"

Sure, it feels like you're getting a bargain because you're getting proportionately more food for proportionately less money. But a "value meal" is only a value for two sets of people: the corporations that make the food and the corporations that make liposuction machines and heart stents. Because food is so inexpensive for manufacturers to produce on a large scale, your average fast-food emporium makes a hefty profit whenever you supersize your meal—even though you're getting an average of 73 percent more calories for only 17 percent more money.

But as we pointed out in the introduction to this book, you're not actually buying more food. You're buying more calories. And that's not something you want more of. (If we were really smart, fast-food shops would be charging us more for the smaller portions!)

IT ALL TASTES THE SAME FOR A REASON

Ever notice how different parts of a fast-food meal kinda taste the same? The burger, the fries, the onion rings, even the shake—they all taste like "fast food." That's because they're all calibrated to appeal to our tastebuds in a way that inspires us to keep eating— not too meaty, not too vegetable-like. The part of our brains called the hypothalamus that responds to food evolved to crave a variety of sweet, salty, and bitter tastes, so we would munch on a variety of foods.

But fast food is designed to satisfy all of these taste desires, so you never crave anything else (like a grapefruit, for example).

KNOW YOUR FOOD

Once upon a time, back when Ray Kroc was still pushing milk-shake machines, a hamburger and fries meant a wad of freshly ground chuck and a peeled, sliced, and fried potato. Now, these two iconic foods—like nearly everything we consume—has taken on a whole new meaning. Sadly, many of our favorite foods today (especially fast foods) weren't merely crafted in kitchens, they were also designed and perfected in labs. So before you mindlessly chew your way through another value meal, visit eatthis.com and search for your favorite restaurant. It'll tell you exactly what you're eating—and which foods to avoid.

Chapter

7

Eat This, Not That!
At Your Supermarket

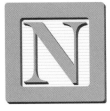EWSFLASH: Your baby's first food won't be mother's milk, applesauce, or Gerber mashed peas, gently spoon-fed into her adorable little rosebud mouth. No, instead, it'll be that box of Oreos you're eating right now. Or the Ezekiel Bread you toasted this morning. Or the Prego sauce and Ronzoni pasta you're planning to serve tonight.

Your baby is taking in—even tasting—the foods you eat, when they're broken down and absorbed in your bloodstream. If you weren't brand-conscious before getting pregnant, you should be now.

Aisle Be There For You

Decoding which brands to trust—and which varieties of those brands to buy—has been the mission of *Eat This, Not That!* for the past decade. And thank goodness. Because unless you understand how food marketers have altered the reality of our weekly trips to the supermarket, it's sometimes impossible to tell what's healthy and what's "healthy."

See, the food industry spends $30 billion a year on advertising—70 percent of it pitching convenience foods, candy, sodas, and desserts. But the real story is this: The food we consume today is different from the food that moms-to-be ate 30 years ago. And the reasons for that are as simple as they are sneaky.

They've Added Extra Calories to Our Food

In the early 1970s, food manufacturers, looking for a cheaper ingredient to replace sugar, came up with a substance called high-fructose corn syrup. Today, HFCS is in an unbelievable array of foods—everything from breakfast cereals to bread, from ketchup to pasta sauce, from juice boxes to iced teas. So Grandma's pasta sauce now comes in a jar, and it's loaded with the stuff.

They've Trained Us to Supersize It

It seems like Economics 101: If you can get a lot more food for just a few cents more, then it makes all the sense in the world to upgrade to the "value meal." And since this trick has worked so well for fast-food marketers, your average product in the supermarket has become Hulkified as well.

They've Laced Our Food with Bad Fats

Most baked goods require oils, and oil leaks at room temperature. But since the 1960s, manufacturers have been baking with something called trans fats. Trans fats are cheap and effective: They make potato chips crispier and cookies tastier. The downside: Trans fats increase your bad cholesterol, lower your good cholesterol, and increase your risk of heart disease.

It's scary. Yet the supermarket is a fact of everyone's life. The average American makes about 1.7 trips a week, and each one of those trips is a chance to eat right, or not. To save money, or to waste it. To set yourself and your baby up for a lifetime of better health, or to deprive you all of the vital nutrients your bodies need to stay strong.

That's why this chapter is designed to make shopping faster, easier, and, most important of all, healthier for you and your baby.

3 Save-Money Shopping Tips

Avoid Quickies

A study supported by the Marketing Science Institute found that shoppers who made "quick trips" to the store purchased an average of 54 percent more merchandise than they had planned to. Instead, be thoughtful in your planning—keep a magnetic notepad on your fridge and make notes throughout the week about what you need.

Bulk Up

Discount clubs are great cost-saving alternatives, even if you have to pay a fee to join. It doesn't make sense to buy everything in bulk, of course—nobody needs a 2-gallon drum of capers. Focus on items you use a lot of and that won't spoil. Cha-ching!

Eat Before You Shop

This is critical! A study published in the *Journal of Consumer Research* found that consumers, even when on a tight budget, are more likely to spend more if their appetites are stimulated before making a purchase. You just know the guys who run the bake shop at the supermarket have read this study too!

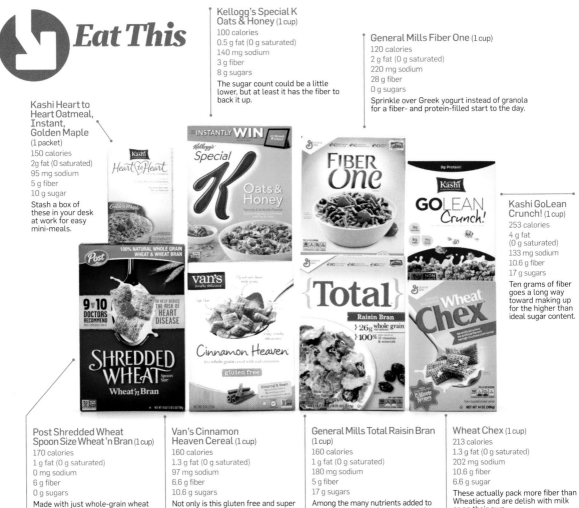

Eat This

Kellogg's Special K Oats & Honey (1 cup)
100 calories
0.5 g fat (0 g saturated)
140 mg sodium
3 g fiber
8 g sugars

The sugar count could be a little lower, but at least it has the fiber to back it up.

General Mills Fiber One (1 cup)
120 calories
2 g fat (0 g saturated)
220 mg sodium
28 g fiber
0 g sugars

Sprinkle over Greek yogurt instead of granola for a fiber- and protein-filled start to the day.

Kashi Heart to Heart Oatmeal, Instant, Golden Maple (1 packet)
150 calories
2 g fat (0 saturated)
95 mg sodium
5 g fiber
10 g sugar

Stash a box of these in your desk at work for easy mini-meals.

Kashi GoLean Crunch! (1 cup)
253 calories
4 g fat (0 g saturated)
133 mg sodium
10.6 g fiber
17 g sugars

Ten grams of fiber goes a long way toward making up for the higher than ideal sugar content.

Post Shredded Wheat Spoon Size Wheat 'n Bran (1 cup)
170 calories
1 g fat (0 g saturated)
0 mg sodium
6 g fiber
0 g sugars

Made with just whole-grain wheat and wheat bran—a pure base crying out for fresh blueberries or bananas.

Van's Cinnamon Heaven Cereal (1 cup)
160 calories
1.3 g fat (0 g saturated)
97 mg sodium
6.6 g fiber
10.6 g sugars

Not only is this gluten free and super good for you, but the cinnamon can help reduce puffiness. Score!

General Mills Total Raisin Bran (1 cup)
160 calories
1 g fat (0 g saturated)
180 mg sodium
5 g fiber
17 g sugars

Among the many nutrients added to each serving in this box are an entire day's worth of calcium and vitamin E.

Wheat Chex (1 cup)
213 calories
1.3 g fat (0 g saturated)
202 mg sodium
10.6 g fiber
6.6 g sugar

These actually pack more fiber than Wheaties and are delish with milk or on their own.

eals

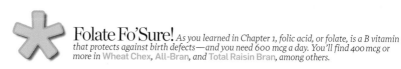

Folate Fo'Sure! *As you learned in Chapter 1, folic acid, or folate, is a B vitamin that protects against birth defects—and you need 600 mcg a day. You'll find 400 mcg or more in Wheat Chex, All-Bran, and Total Raisin Bran, among others.*

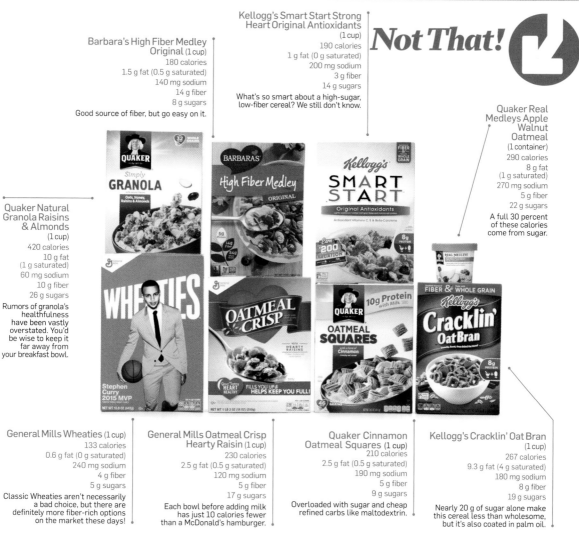

Kellogg's Smart Start Strong Heart Original Antioxidants
(1 cup)
190 calories
1 g fat (0 g saturated)
200 mg sodium
3 g fiber
14 g sugars

What's so smart about a high-sugar, low-fiber cereal? We still don't know.

Not That!

Barbara's High Fiber Medley Original (1 cup)
180 calories
1.5 g fat (0.5 g saturated)
140 mg sodium
14 g fiber
8 g sugars
Good source of fiber, but go easy on it.

Quaker Real Medleys Apple Walnut Oatmeal
(1 container)
290 calories
8 g fat
(1 g saturated)
270 mg sodium
5 g fiber
22 g sugars
A full 30 percent of these calories come from sugar.

Quaker Natural Granola Raisins & Almonds
(1 cup)
420 calories
10 g fat
(1 g saturated)
60 mg sodium
10 g fiber
26 g sugars
Rumors of granola's healthfulness have been vastly overstated. You'd be wise to keep it far away from your breakfast bowl.

General Mills Wheaties (1 cup)
133 calories
0.6 g fat (0 g saturated)
240 mg sodium
4 g fiber
5 g sugars
Classic Wheaties aren't necessarily a bad choice, but there are definitely more fiber-rich options on the market these days!

General Mills Oatmeal Crisp Hearty Raisin (1 cup)
230 calories
2.5 g fat (0.5 g saturated)
120 mg sodium
5 g fiber
17 g sugars
Each bowl before adding milk has just 10 calories fewer than a McDonald's hamburger.

Quaker Cinnamon Oatmeal Squares (1 cup)
210 calories
2.5 g fat (0.5 g saturated)
190 mg sodium
5 g fiber
9 g sugars
Overloaded with sugar and cheap refined carbs like maltodextrin.

Kellogg's Cracklin' Oat Bran (1 cup)
267 calories
9.3 g fat (4 g saturated)
180 mg sodium
8 g fiber
19 g sugars
Nearly 20 g of sugar alone make this cereal less than wholesome, but it's also coated in palm oil.

Breakfast Breads

Eat This

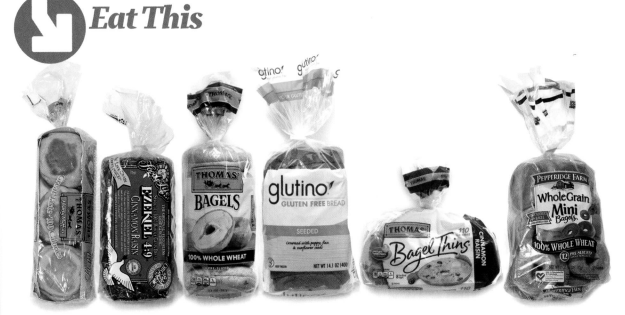

Thomas' Light Multi-Grain English Muffins
1 muffin, 57 g
100 calories
1 g fat (0 g saturated)
160 mg sodium
26 g carbohydrates
8 g fiber

Outside of green vegetables, you'll find very few foods that pack 8 grams of fiber into 100 calories. That makes this an unbeatable foundation for breakfast sandwiches.

Food for Life Ezekiel 4:9 Sprouted 100% Whole Grain Cinnamon Raisin Bread
(1 slice, 34 g)
80 calories
0 g fat (0 g saturated)
65 mg sodium
18 g carbohydrates
2 g fiber

Barley, millet, and spelt help boost fiber.

Thomas' 100% Whole Wheat Bagels
(1 bagel, 95 g)
240 calories
2 g fat (0.5 g saturated)
400 mg sodium
49 g carbohydrates
7 g fiber

A bagel that packs a whopping 10 grams of protein? Sign. Us. Up.

Glutino Seeded Bread
(1 slice, 29 g)
80 calories
3 g fat (0 g saturated)
170 mg sodium
13 g carbohydrates
7 g fiber

Sunflower, flax, and poppy seeds give this bread a decent hit of healthy fats for hardly any calories.

Thomas' Bagel Thins Cinnamon Raisin
(1 bagel, 46 g)
110 calories
1 g fat (0 g saturated)
160 mg sodium
25 g carbohydrates
5 g fiber

Switching to these is the best way to wean yourself off bagels. Try a swipe of peanut butter instead of cream cheese for a near-perfect snack.

Pepperidge Farm Whole Grain Mini Bagels 100% Whole Wheat
(1 bagel, 40 g)
100 calories
0.5 g fat (0 g saturated)
120 mg sodium
20 g carbohydrates
3 g fiber

The perfect base for a ham and egg breakfast sandwich.

THE WHOLE TRUTH
You want breads labeled "whole grain" or "whole wheat." Not "wheat flour."

FREEZE!
Can't find a healthy carb in the bread aisle? Check the frozen foods section for a sprouted grain bread, like Ezekiel.

Not That!

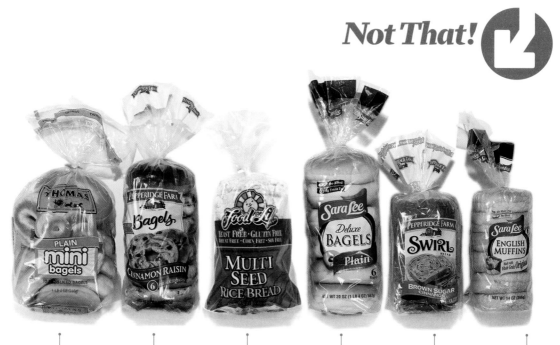

Thomas' Plain Mini Bagels
(1 bagel, 43 g)
120 calories
1 g fat (0 g saturated)
210 mg sodium
24 g carbohydrates
1 g fiber

Once your palate is accustomed to whole grains, flavorless, nutritionless lumps of refined carbs like this will taste boring.

Pepperidge Farm Bagels Cinnamon Raisin
(1 bagel, 99 g)
270 calories
1 g fat (0 g saturated)
290 mg sodium
57 g carbohydrates
3 g fiber

This bagel belongs on a dessert menu, not a breakfast table.

Food for Life Gluten-Free Multi-Seed Rice Bread
(1 slice, 50g)
120 calories
1 g fat (0 g saturated)
170 mg sodium
26 g carbohydrates
1 g fiber

What this rice-and-tapioca concoction cuts in gluten it doesn't make up for in whole grains.

Sara Lee Deluxe Bagels Plain
(1 bagel, 95 g)
260 calories
1 g fat (0 g saturated)
400 mg sodium
50 g carbohydrates
2 g fiber

This is a wedge of refined carbohydrates, and as such, it will induce a blood sugar roller coaster that will wreak havoc on your energy reserves.

Pepperidge Farm Brown Sugar Cinnamon Swirl Bread
(1 slice, 38 g)
80 calories
1.5 g fat (0 g saturated)
110 mg sodium
15 g carbohydrates
<1 g fiber

This bread contains four different forms of sugar.

Sara Lee Original Made with Whole Grain English Muffins
1 muffin, 66 g
140 calories
1 g fat (0 g saturated)
210 mg sodium
27 g carbohydrates
2 g fiber

The more fiber you work into your breakfast, the more likely you'll be to make it to lunch without experiencing hunger pangs. That means this muffin is a recipe for midmorning cravings.

219

Yogurts

Eat This

Chobani Greek Yogurt Simply 100 Strawberry
(1 container, 5.3 oz)
100 calories
0 g fat (0 g saturated)
5 g fiber
7 g sugars
12 g protein

There's a reason why Chobani has become the yogurt of the moment. With nearly three times the protein, half the sugar, and way more fiber than most fat-free brands, it's a clear winner.

YoCrunch Parfait Strawberry
(1 container, 4 oz)
110 calories
0.5 g fat (0 g saturated)
<1g fiber
16 g sugar
3 g protein

Impressively low-cal for a fruity, crunchy parfait. Get your crunch on!

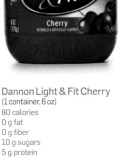

Dannon Oikos Greek Nonfat Yogurt
(1 container, 5.3 oz)
80 calories
0 g fat (0 g saturated)
0 g fiber
6 g sugar
15 g protein

Enjoy this every day—it's got the highest-protein count on this page!

Dannon Light & Fit Cherry
(1 container, 6 oz)
80 calories
0 g fat
0 g fiber
10 g sugars
5 g protein

We prefer a yogurt with more protein, but it's tough to argue against one with just 80 calories per serving.

Siggi's Icelandic Style Skyr Strained Non Fat Yogurt Vanilla
(1 container, 5.3 oz)
100 calories
0 g fat
0 g fiber
9 g sugars
14 g protein

Strained just like Greek yogurt, which makes it creamy and high-protein.

Lifeway Lowfat Kefir Strawberry
(1 container, 8 oz)
140 calories
2 g fat (1.5 g saturated)
20 g sugars
11 g protein

Kefir is 99 percent lactose free, making it suitable for most intolerant individuals. It also happens to be a stellar source of protein and probiotic bacteria.

✚ YO GIRL!

Make sure that your yogurt comes in a container marked 1, 2, 4, or 5 (check the bottom)—those have no BPA, a chemical linked to belly fat.

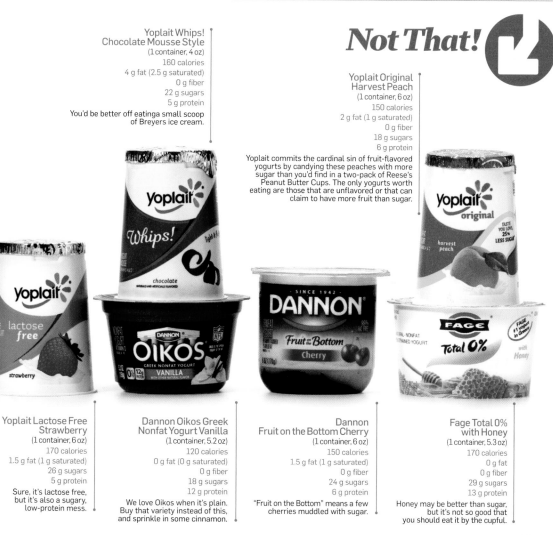

Yoplait Whips! Chocolate Mousse Style
(1 container, 4 oz)
160 calories
4 g fat (2.5 g saturated)
0 g fiber
22 g sugars
5 g protein

You'd be better off eatinga small scoop of Breyers ice cream.

Not That!

Yoplait Original Harvest Peach
(1 container, 6 oz)
150 calories
2 g fat (1 g saturated)
0 g fiber
18 g sugars
6 g protein

Yoplait commits the cardinal sin of fruit-flavored yogurts by candying these peaches with more sugar than you'd find in a two-pack of Reese's Peanut Butter Cups. The only yogurts worth eating are those that are unflavored or that can claim to have more fruit than sugar.

Yoplait Lactose Free Strawberry
(1 container, 6 oz)
170 calories
1.5 g fat (1 g saturated)
26 g sugars
5 g protein

Sure, it's lactose free, but it's also a sugary, low-protein mess.

Dannon Oikos Greek Nonfat Yogurt Vanilla
(1 container, 5.2 oz)
120 calories
0 g fat (0 g saturated)
0 g fiber
18 g sugars
12 g protein

We love Oikos when it's plain. Buy that variety instead of this, and sprinkle in some cinnamon.

Dannon Fruit on the Bottom Cherry
(1 container, 6 oz)
150 calories
1.5 g fat (1 g saturated)
0 g fiber
24 g sugars
6 g protein

"Fruit on the Bottom" means a few cherries muddled with sugar.

Fage Total 0% with Honey
(1 container, 5.3 oz)
170 calories
0 g fat
0 g fiber
29 g sugars
13 g protein

Honey may be better than sugar, but it's not so good that you should eat it by the cupful.

Cheeses

Eat This

Kraft Singles 2% Milk Sharp Cheddar
(1 slice, 21 g)
60 calories
4 g fat (2.5 g saturated)
240 mg sodium
4 g protein

There may be a few lighter cheeses out there, but they don't taste like cheese. If you're looking for an all-purpose burger or sandwich topper, start here.

The Laughing Cow Original Creamy Swiss
(1 wedge, 21 g)
50 calories
4 g fat (2.5 g saturated)
190 mg sodium
2 g protein

Spreads every bit as easily as Alouette's, yet it cuts your calorie load by a third.

Bel Gioioso Sliced Mozzarella
(1 oz, 28 g)
70 calories
5 g fat (3 g saturated)
85 mg sodium
5 g protein

Made with hormone-free milk, this creamy snack boasts automatic portion control and lower sodium than other brands.

Athenos Traditional Crumbled Feta
(¼ cup, 28 g)
70 calories
6 g fat (3.5 g saturated)
330 mg sodium
5 g protein

A reasonable fat-to-protein ratio makes feta the most reliable go-to pasteurized cheese.

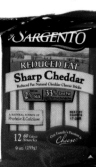
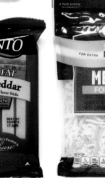
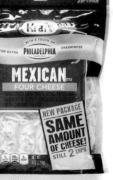
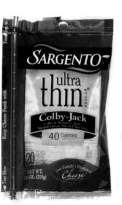
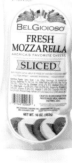

Cabot 50% Reduced Fat Sharp Cheddar
(1" cube, 28 g)
70 calories
4.5 g fat (3 g saturated)
170 mg sodium
8 g protein

A smart approach: Cut half the fat but leave enough to add a rich, creamy texture.

Sargento Reduced Fat Sharp Cheddar Sticks
(1 stick, 21 g)
60 calories
4.5 g fat (3 g saturated)
135 mg sodium
5 g protein

Portable snacks don't get any better than this.

Kraft Natural Mexican Style Queso Quesadilla with a Touch of Philadelphia
(¼ cup, 28 g)
90 calories
7 g fat (4 g saturated)
160 mg sodium
6 g protein

An unusually low-cal cheese blend.

Sargento Ultra Thin Colby Jack
(2 slices, 21 g)
86 calories
6.6 g fat (4.6 g saturated)
146 mg sodium
5.3 g protein

Sargento's thinner slices cut calories without sacrificing any flavor.

Should You Cut the Cheese?

Most cheeses in U.S. supermarkets—even soft ones like brie, feta, and goat cheese—are pasteurized, meaning they're safe for you and baby. Just be sure to read labels and avoid anything unpasteurized!

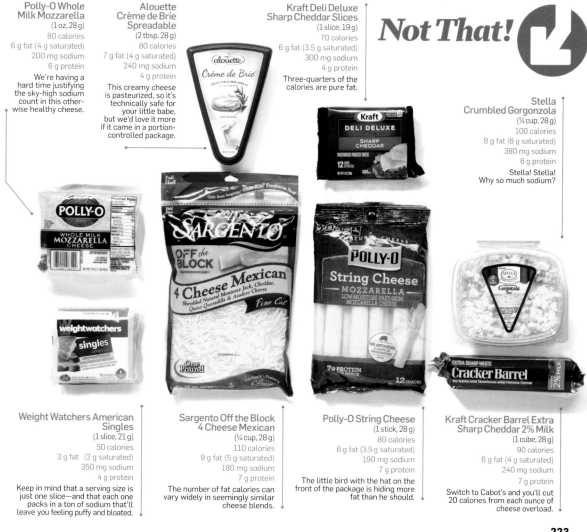

Polly-O Whole Milk Mozzarella
(1 oz, 28 g)
80 calories
6 g fat (4 g saturated)
200 mg sodium
6 g protein

We're having a hard time justifying the sky-high sodium count in this otherwise healthy cheese.

Alouette Crème de Brie Spreadable
(2 tbsp, 28 g)
80 calories
7 g fat (4 g saturated)
240 mg sodium
4 g protein

This creamy cheese is pasteurized, so it's technically safe for your little babe, but we'd love it more if it came in a portion-controlled package.

Kraft Deli Deluxe Sharp Cheddar Slices
(1 slice, 19 g)
70 calories
6 g fat (3.5 g saturated)
300 mg sodium
4 g protein

Three-quarters of the calories are pure fat.

Not That!

Stella Crumbled Gorgonzola
(¼ cup, 28 g)
100 calories
8 g fat (6 g saturated)
380 mg sodium
6 g protein

Stella! Stella! Why so much sodium?

Weight Watchers American Singles
(1 slice, 21 g)
50 calories
3 g fat (2 g saturated)
350 mg sodium
4 g protein

Keep in mind that a serving size is just one slice—and that each one packs in a ton of sodium that'll leave you feeling puffy and bloated.

Sargento Off the Block 4 Cheese Mexican
(¼ cup, 28 g)
110 calories
9 g fat (5 g saturated)
180 mg sodium
7 g protein

The number of fat calories can vary widely in seemingly similar cheese blends.

Polly-O String Cheese
(1 stick, 28 g)
80 calories
6 g fat (3.5 g saturated)
190 mg sodium
7 g protein

The little bird with the hat on the front of the package is hiding more fat than he should.

Kraft Cracker Barrel Extra Sharp Cheddar 2% Milk
(1 cube, 28 g)
90 calories
6 g fat (4 g saturated)
240 mg sodium
7 g protein

Switch to Cabot's and you'll cut 20 calories from each ounce of cheese overload.

Deli Meats

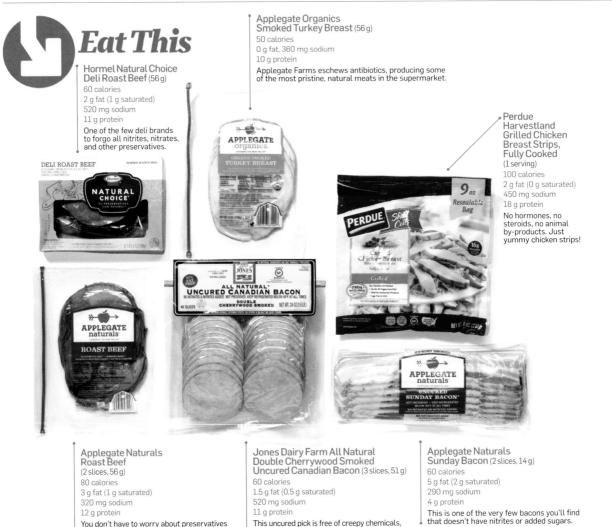

Applegate Organics Smoked Turkey Breast (56 g)

50 calories
0 g fat, 360 mg sodium
10 g protein

Applegate Farms eschews antibiotics, producing some of the most pristine, natural meats in the supermarket.

Hormel Natural Choice Deli Roast Beef (56 g)

60 calories
2 g fat (1 g saturated)
520 mg sodium
11 g protein

One of the few deli brands to forgo all nitrites, nitrates, and other preservatives.

Perdue Harvestland Grilled Chicken Breast Strips, Fully Cooked

(1 serving)
100 calories
2 g fat (0 g saturated)
450 mg sodium
18 g protein

No hormones, no steroids, no animal by-products. Just yummy chicken strips!

Applegate Naturals Roast Beef

(2 slices, 56 g)
80 calories
3 g fat (1 g saturated)
320 mg sodium
12 g protein

You don't have to worry about preservatives or added nitrites with this choice!

Jones Dairy Farm All Natural Double Cherrywood Smoked Uncured Canadian Bacon (3 slices, 51 g)

60 calories
1.5 g fat (0.5 g saturated)
520 mg sodium
11 g protein

This uncured pick is free of creepy chemicals, but full of the healthy protein you crave.

Applegate Naturals Sunday Bacon (2 slices, 14 g)

60 calories
5 g fat (2 g saturated)
290 mg sodium
4 g protein

This is one of the very few bacons you'll find that doesn't have nitrites or added sugars.

HEAT IT UP!

Deli meats are responsible for 85% of all pregnancy-threatening Listeria cases. But if you always heat them before eating—and only keep deli meats at home for five days after they've been opened—they're fine to eat.

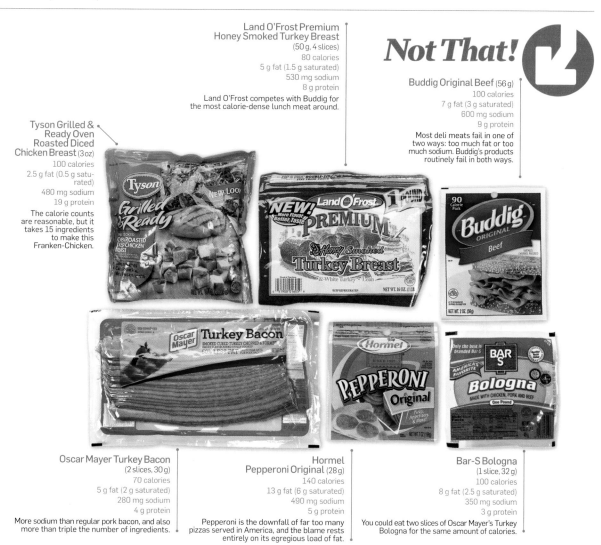

Land O'Frost Premium Honey Smoked Turkey Breast
(50 g, 4 slices)
80 calories
5 g fat (1.5 g saturated)
530 mg sodium
8 g protein

Land O'Frost competes with Buddig for the most calorie-dense lunch meat around.

Not That!

Buddig Original Beef (56 g)
100 calories
7 g fat (3 g saturated)
600 mg sodium
9 g protein

Most deli meats fail in one of two ways: too much fat or too much sodium. Buddig's products routinely fail in both ways.

Tyson Grilled & Ready Oven Roasted Diced Chicken Breast (3 oz)
100 calories
2.5 g fat (0.5 g saturated)
480 mg sodium
19 g protein

The calorie counts are reasonable, but it takes 15 ingredients to make this Franken-Chicken.

Oscar Mayer Turkey Bacon
(2 slices, 30 g)
70 calories
5 g fat (2 g saturated)
280 mg sodium
4 g protein

More sodium than regular pork bacon, and also more than triple the number of ingredients.

Hormel Pepperoni Original (28 g)
140 calories
13 g fat (6 g saturated)
490 mg sodium
5 g protein

Pepperoni is the downfall of far too many pizzas served in America, and the blame rests entirely on its egregious load of fat.

Bar-S Bologna
(1 slice, 32 g)
100 calories
8 g fat (2.5 g saturated)
350 mg sodium
3 g protein

You could eat two slices of Oscar Mayer's Turkey Bologna for the same amount of calories.

Condiments

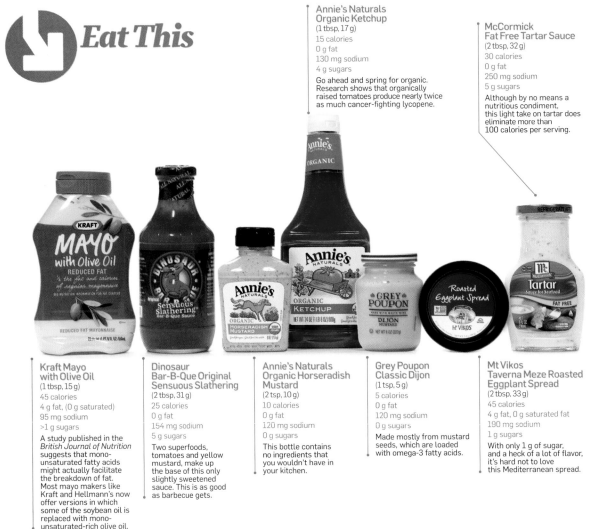

Eat This

Annie's Naturals Organic Ketchup
(1 tbsp, 17 g)
15 calories
0 g fat
130 mg sodium
4 g sugars

Go ahead and spring for organic. Research shows that organically raised tomatoes produce nearly twice as much cancer-fighting lycopene.

McCormick Fat Free Tartar Sauce
(2 tbsp, 32 g)
30 calories
0 g fat
250 mg sodium
5 g sugars

Although by no means a nutritious condiment, this light take on tartar does eliminate more than 100 calories per serving.

Kraft Mayo with Olive Oil
(1 tbsp, 15 g)
45 calories
4 g fat, (0 g saturated)
95 mg sodium
>1 g sugars

A study published in the *British Journal of Nutrition* suggests that mono-unsaturated fatty acids might actually facilitate the breakdown of fat. Most mayo makers like Kraft and Hellmann's now offer versions in which some of the soybean oil is replaced with mono-unsaturated-rich olive oil.

Dinosaur Bar-B-Que Original Sensuous Slathering
(2 tbsp, 31 g)
25 calories
0 g fat
154 mg sodium
5 g sugars

Two superfoods, tomatoes and yellow mustard, make up the base of this only slightly sweetened sauce. This is as good as barbecue gets.

Annie's Naturals Organic Horseradish Mustard
(2 tsp, 10 g)
10 calories
0 g fat
120 mg sodium
0 g sugars

This bottle contains no ingredients that you wouldn't have in your kitchen.

Grey Poupon Classic Dijon
(1 tsp, 5 g)
5 calories
0 g fat
120 mg sodium
0 g sugars

Made mostly from mustard seeds, which are loaded with omega-3 fatty acids.

Mt Vikos Taverna Meze Roasted Eggplant Spread
(2 tbsp, 33 g)
45 calories
4 g fat, 0 g saturated fat
190 mg sodium
1 g sugars

With only 1 g of sugar, and a heck of a lot of flavor, it's hard not to love this Mediterranean spread.

226

The main ingredient in many sauces is high-fructose corn syrup. Avoid them. That provides an excessive sugar load, unecessary because the vegetable-base provides flavor enough.

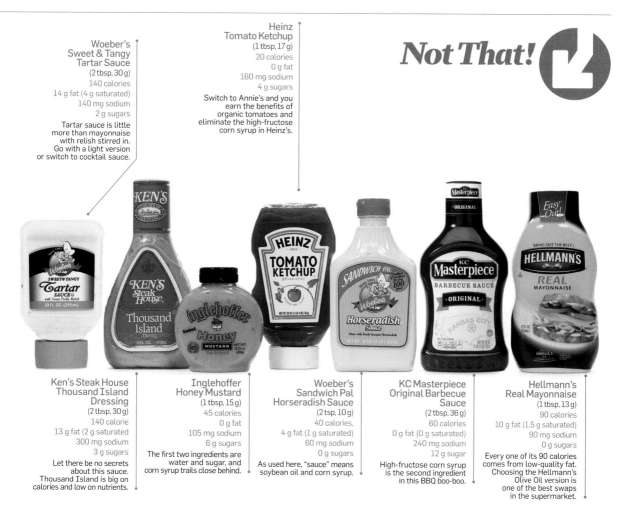

Not That!

**Woeber's
Sweet & Tangy
Tartar Sauce**
(2 tbsp, 30 g)
140 calories
14 g fat (4 g saturated)
140 mg sodium
2 g sugars

Tartar sauce is little
more than mayonnaise
with relish stirred in.
Go with a light version
or switch to cocktail sauce.

**Heinz
Tomato Ketchup**
(1 tbsp, 17 g)
20 calories
0 g fat
160 mg sodium
4 g sugars

Switch to Annie's and you
earn the benefits of
organic tomatoes and
eliminate the high-fructose
corn syrup in Heinz's.

**Ken's Steak House
Thousand Island
Dressing**
(2 tbsp, 30 g)
140 calorie
13 g fat (2 g saturated)
300 mg sodium
3 g sugars

Let there be no secrets
about this sauce.
Thousand Island is big on
calories and low on nutrients.

**Inglehoffer
Honey Mustard**
(1 tbsp, 15 g)
45 calories
0 g fat
105 mg sodium
6 g sugars

The first two ingredients are
water and sugar, and
corn syrup trails close behind.

**Woeber's
Sandwich Pal
Horseradish Sauce**
(2 tsp, 10 g)
40 calories,
4 g fat (1 g saturated)
60 mg sodium
0 g sugars

As used here, "sauce" means
soybean oil and corn syrup.

**KC Masterpiece
Original Barbecue
Sauce**
(2 tbsp, 36 g)
60 calories
0 g fat (0 g saturated)
240 mg sodium
12 g sugar

High-fructose corn syrup
is the second ingredient
in this BBQ boo-boo.

**Hellmann's
Real Mayonnaise**
(1 tbsp, 13 g)
90 calories
10 g fat (1.5 g saturated)
90 mg sodium
0 g sugars

Every one of its 90 calories
comes from low-quality fat.
Choosing the Hellmann's
Olive Oil version is
one of the best swaps
in the supermarket.

Breads

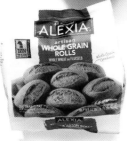

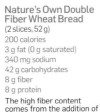

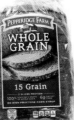

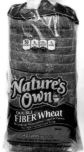

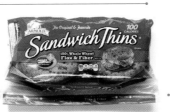

Eat This

Nature's Own Double Fiber Wheat Bread
(2 slices, 52 g)
200 calories
3 g fat (0 g saturated)
340 mg sodium
42 g carbohydrates
8 g fiber
8 g protein

The high fiber content comes from the addition of inulin, a natural fiber made from chicory.

Pepperidge Farm Whole Grain 15 Grain
(2 slices, 86 g)
220 calories
4 g fat (1 g saturated)
250 mg sodium
40 g carbohydrates
6 g fiber
10 g protein

Five grams of protein and 4 grams of fiber per slice? Yes, please!

Arnold Sandwich Thins Flax & Fiber
(1 roll, 43 g)
100 calories
1 g fat (0 g saturated)
170 mg sodium
21 g carbohydrates
5 g fiber
5 g protein

Protein and fiber supply more than a third of these calories.

Alexia Artisan Whole Grain Rolls
(1 roll, 43 g)
110 calories
1 g fat (0 g saturated)
190 mg sodium
19 g carbohydrates
3 g fiber
6 g protein

If your roll is over 100 calories, it had better have a hefty amount of protein—and this one does!

Mission Yellow Extra Thin Corn Tortillas
(2 tortillas, 37 g)
72 calories
1 g fat (0 g saturated)
6 mg sodium
14.5 g carbohydrates
3 g fiber
2 g protein

Fiber-rich corn trumps flour every time in the tortilla battle.

Martin's 100% Whole Wheat Potato Rolls
(1 roll, 42.5 g)
100 calories
1.5 g fat (0 g saturated)
150 mg sodium
18 g carbohydrates
3 g fiber
7 g protein

A perfect burger bun. Whole wheat adds a potent fiber punch.

Flatout Light Original Flatbread
(1 piece, 53 g)
90 calories
1.5 g fat (0 g saturated)
250 mg sodium
14 g carbohydrates
8 g fiber
9 g protein

Not one of Flatout's flatbreads has fewer than 3 grams of fiber.

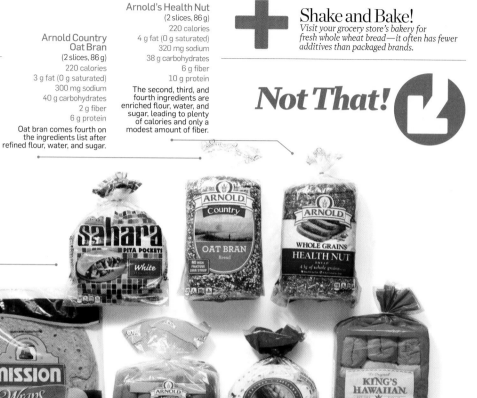

Arnold's Health Nut
(2 slices, 86 g)
220 calories
4 g fat (0 g saturated)
320 mg sodium
38 g carbohydrates
6 g fiber
10 g protein

The second, third, and fourth ingredients are enriched flour, water, and sugar, leading to plenty of calories and only a modest amount of fiber.

Arnold Country Oat Bran
(2 slices, 86 g)
220 calories
3 g fat (0 g saturated)
300 mg sodium
40 g carbohydrates
2 g fiber
6 g protein

Oat bran comes fourth on the ingredients list after refined flour, water, and sugar.

Shake and Bake!

Visit your grocery store's bakery for fresh whole wheat bread—it often has fewer additives than packaged brands.

Not That!

Thomas' Sahara Pita Bread White
(1 pita, 57 g)
160 calories
1.5 g fat (0 g saturated)
250 mg sodium
31 g carbohydrates
1 g fiber
6 g protein

Switch to a pita with fewer carbs and use the saved calories to double up on hummus!

Mission Wraps Garden Spinach Herb
(1 wrap, 70 g)
210 calories
5 g fat (2 g saturated)
440 mg sodium
36 g carbohydrates
3 g fiber
6 g protein

The only spinach here is "spinach powder," which accounts for less than 2 percent of each wrap.

Arnold Potato Hot Dog Rolls
(1 roll, 76 g)
140 calories
1 g fat (0 g saturated)
280 mg sodium
27 g carbohydrates
1 g fiber
5 g protein

Like most rolls, these are just pillows of empty carbs.

Guerrero Soft Taco Homemade Flour Tortillas
(1 tortilla, 37 g)
100 calories
3.5 g fat (1.5 g saturated)
260 mg sodium
15 g carbohydrates
2 g fiber
3 g protein

It takes more than 15 ingredients to construct this tortured tortilla.

King's Hawaiian Original Hawaiian Sweet Rolls
(1 roll, 28 g)
90 calories
2 g fat (1 g saturated)
80 mg sodium
16 g carbohydrates
0 g fiber
3 g protein

Why would you put these on your table when they've got zero fiber?

Grains & Noodles

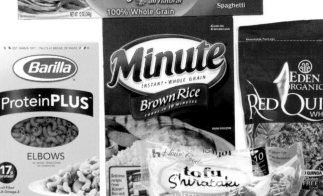
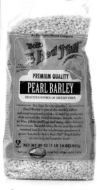

Eat This

Ronzoni Healthy Harvest Whole Grain Spaghetti
(2 oz, 56 g dry)

180 calories
1.5 g fat (0 g saturated)
39 g carbohydrates
5 g fiber

Whole-grain pastas are loaded with fiber, and diets rich in fiber are shown to decrease your odds of developing both diabetes and heart disease. You want about 20 grams per day, and this spaghetti has 30 percent of that.

Eden Organic Red Quinoa
(¼ cup, 45 g dry)

170 calories
2 g fat (0 g saturated)
32 g carbohydrates
5 g fiber

Quinoa contains every amino acid your body needs from food. That's a claim rice can't make.

Barilla ProteinPLUS Elbows
(56 g dry)

190 calories
2 g fat (0 g saturated)
38 g carbohydrates
4 g fiber

Whole grain pastas are loaded with fiber, which will keep you feeling fuller longer and help you avoid feeling stopped up. Plus? This amazing pasta packs 10 g of protein and is a good source of iron, too!

Minute Brown Rice
(½ cup, 50 g dry)

180 calories
1.5 g fat (0 g saturated)
39 g carbohydrates
2 g fiber

Eating healthy doesn't take more time; it just requires being more strategic in the supermarket.

House Foods Tofu Shirataki Spaghetti
(113 g)

10 calories
0.5 g fat (0 g saturated)
3 g carbohydrates
2 g fiber

These traditional Asian noodles are made from tofu and yam flour. Don't be afraid—they have a neutral flavor that's perfect for dressing up.

Bob's Red Mill Pearl Barley
(¼ cup, 50 g dry)

180 calories
1 g fat (0 g saturated)
39 g carbohydrates
8 g fiber

Perfect for adding nutritional heft to everyday soups. Try using it as a replacement for noodles in minestrone.

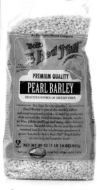

BROWN BAG IT

Eating whole grains and brown pastas fill you up more than the refined stuff, but also lower blood pressure.

MRS. BEAN!

To boost belly-filling fiber, opt for a bean-based noodle such as Banza Chickpea Shells.

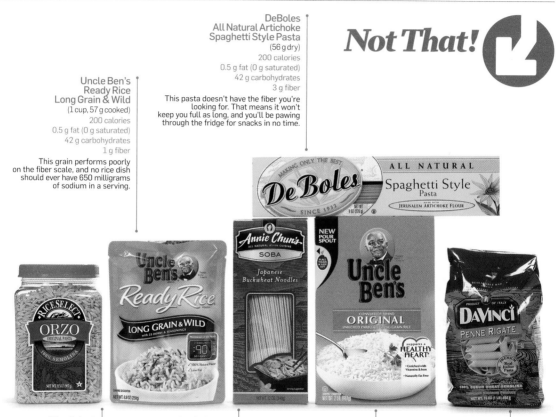

**DeBoles
All Natural Artichoke
Spaghetti Style Pasta**
(56 g dry)
200 calories
0.5 g fat (0 g saturated)
42 g carbohydrates
3 g fiber

This pasta doesn't have the fiber you're looking for. That means it won't keep you full as long, and you'll be pawing through the fridge for snacks in no time.

Not That!

**Uncle Ben's
Ready Rice
Long Grain & Wild**
(1 cup, 57 g cooked)
200 calories
0.5 g fat (0 g saturated)
42 g carbohydrates
1 g fiber

This grain performs poorly on the fiber scale, and no rice dish should ever have 650 milligrams of sodium in a serving.

**RiceSelect
Orzo**
(⅓ cup, 56 g dry)
210 calories
1 g fat (0 g saturated)
42 g carbohydrates
2 g fiber

Essentially, these are little nibs of refined pasta. You're far better off using a legitimate whole grain.

**Annie Chun's
Soba Noodles**
(57 g dry)
200 calories
1 g fat (0 g saturated)
39 g carbohydrates
3 g fiber

Japanese-style soba noodles tend to carry much more salt than Italian pasta noodles. A single serving of these packs 390 milligrams of sodium.

**Uncle Ben's
Original Rice**
(¼ cup, 47 g dry)
170 calories
0 g fat
37 g carbohydrates
0 g fiber

Never eat rice, pasta, or other starchy sides unless they have fiber. Otherwise, they'll spike your blood sugar like a pile of candy.

**DaVinci
Penne Rigate**
(½ cup, 56 g dry)
200 calories
1 g fat (0 g saturated)
41 g carbohydrates
2 g fiber

Healthier noodles are available in all shapes and sizes, so there's never a reason to settle for one that's high in calories and low in fiber like this one is.

231

Sauces

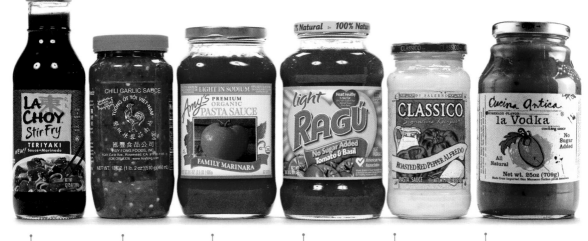

La Choy Teriyaki Stir Fry Sauce & Marinade

(1 tbsp, 16 g)

10 calories

0 g fat

105 mg sodium

1 g sugars

The typical teriyaki sauce suffers from two blights: too much sodium and too much sugar. This one avoids both, which makes it by far the best teriyaki in the supermarket.

Huy Fong Chili Garlic Sauce

(1 tsp, 5 g)

0 calories

0 g fat

95 mg sodium

<1 g sugars

Chili pepper is the primary ingredient, and it contains not a single gram of added sugar.

Amy's Light in Sodium Organic Family Marinara

(½ cup)

80 calories,

4.5 g fat
(0.5 g saturated)

290 mg sodium

5 g sugars

Stick with the low-sodium version. Amy's regular marinara has 290 milligrams more sodium.

Ragú Light No Sugar Added Tomato & Basil

(½ cup)

50 calories

0 g fat (0 g saturated)

320 mg sodium

6 g sugars

Think Italians add sugar to their marinara? Of course not—added sugars mask the naturally sweet flavor of cooked tomatoes.

Classico Roasted Red Pepper Alfredo

(½ cup)

120 calories

8 g fat (6 g saturated)

620 mg sodium

2 g sugars

Smart move: The roasted red peppers in this jar displace a heavy load of fatty cream and cheese calories.

Cucina Antica La Vodka

(½ cup)

50 calories

3.5 g fat
(2.5 g saturated)

220 mg sodium

2 g sugars

Cucina Antica gets the tomato-to-cream ratio right with this superlative sauce.

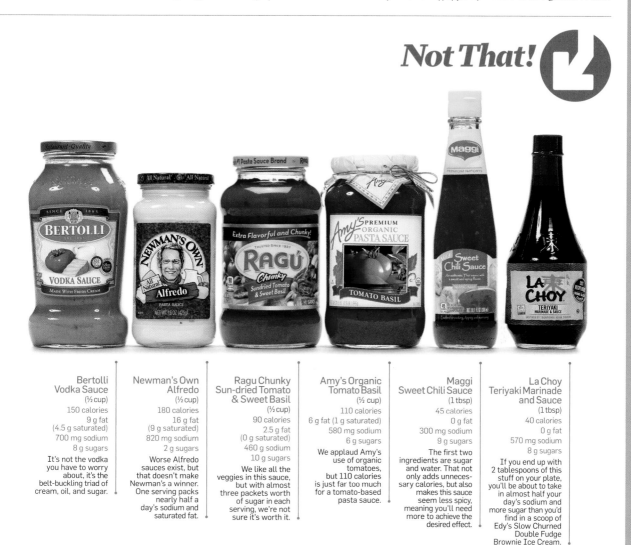

Some sauces contain 14 grams or more of sugar, which means they pack more than a serving of Frosted Flakes! Your baby's better off if you find one with 6 grams or less.

Not That!

Bertolli Vodka Sauce
(½ cup)
150 calories
9 g fat
(4.5 g saturated)
700 mg sodium
8 g sugars

It's not the vodka you have to worry about, it's the belt-buckling triad of cream, oil, and sugar.

Newman's Own Alfredo
(½ cup)
180 calories
16 g fat
(9 g saturated)
820 mg sodium
2 g sugars

Worse Alfredo sauces exist, but that doesn't make Newman's a winner. One serving packs nearly half a day's sodium and saturated fat.

Ragu Chunky Sun-dried Tomato & Sweet Basil
(½ cup)
90 calories
2.5 g fat
(0 g saturated)
460 g sodium
10 g sugars

We like all the veggies in this sauce, but with almost three packets worth of sugar in each serving, we're not sure it's worth it.

Amy's Organic Tomato Basil
(½ cup)
110 calories
6 g fat (1 g saturated)
580 mg sodium
6 g sugars

We applaud Amy's use of organic tomatoes, but 110 calories is just far too much for a tomato-based pasta sauce.

Maggi Sweet Chili Sauce
(1 tbsp)
45 calories
0 g fat
300 mg sodium
9 g sugars

The first two ingredients are sugar and water. That not only adds unnecessary calories, but also makes this sauce seem less spicy, meaning you'll need more to achieve the desired effect.

La Choy Teriyaki Marinade and Sauce
(1 tbsp)
40 calories
0 g fat
570 mg sodium
8 g sugars

If you end up with 2 tablespoons of this stuff on your plate, you'll be about to take in almost half your day's sodium and more sugar than you'd find in a scoop of Edy's Slow Churned Double Fudge Brownie Ice Cream.

Soups

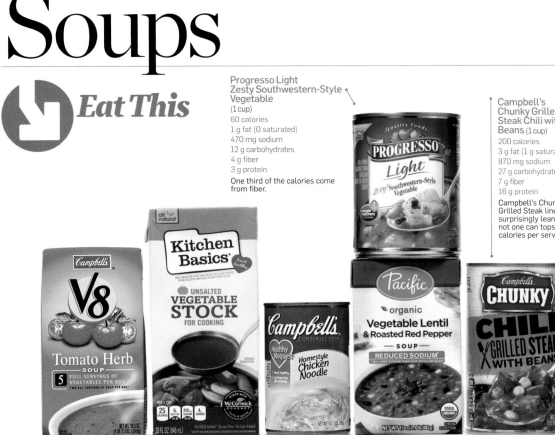

Eat This

Progresso Light Zesty Southwestern-Style Vegetable
(1 cup)
60 calories
1 g fat (0 saturated)
470 mg sodium
12 g carbohydrates
4 g fiber
3 g protein
One third of the calories come from fiber.

Campbell's Chunky Grilled Steak Chili with Beans (1 cup)
200 calories
3 g fat (1 g saturated)
870 mg sodium
27 g carbohydrates
7 g fiber
16 g protein
Campbell's Chunky Grilled Steak line is surprisingly lean—not one can tops 200 calories per serving.

V8 Tomato Herb
(1 cup)
90 calories
0 g fat
480 mg sodium
19 g carbohydrates
3 g fiber
3 g protein
Carrots and red peppers are among the primary ingredients in this carton. That's how each serving earns you nearly half of your daily vitamin A requirement.

Kitchen Basics Unsalted Vegetable Cooking Stock
(1 cup)
25 calories
0 g fat (0 g saturated)
210 mg sodium
6 g carbohydrates
0 g fiber
2 g protein
Whether you're looking for a base for your own homemade soup or for a broth to sip on, this one rates relatively low in sodium, and high on flavor.

Campbell's Healthy Request Condensed Homestyle Chicken Noodle
(½ cup condensed)
60 calories
2 g fat (0.5 saturated)
410 mg sodium
8 g carbohydrates
1 g fiber
3 g protein
Low cal, light sodium.

Pacific Organic Low in Sodium Vegetable Lentil & Roasted Red Pepper Soup
(1 cup)
150 calories
0.5 g fat (0 g saturated)
490 mg sodium
27 g carbohydrates
7 g fiber
8 g protein
Want protein without the meat? The lentils in this hearty soup deliver big time.

SHOULD YOU CAN THE CANS?

While I'd always advise eating homemade soups over their sodium-filled canned cousins, we know sometimes that's just not an option. If you are cracking open a can of hearty soup, make sure the can isn't dented. That could be a sign of botulism.

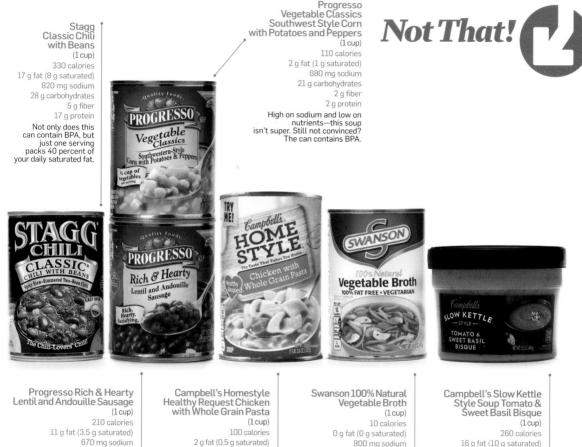

Not That!

Stagg Classic Chili with Beans
(1 cup)
330 calories
17 g fat (8 g saturated)
820 mg sodium
28 g carbohydrates
5 g fiber
17 g protein

Not only does this can contain BPA, but just one serving packs 40 percent of your daily saturated fat.

Progresso Vegetable Classics Southwest Style Corn with Potatoes and Peppers
(1 cup)
110 calories
2 g fat (1 g saturated)
680 mg sodium
21 g carbohydrates
2 g fiber
2 g protein

High on sodium and low on nutrients—this soup isn't super. Still not convinced? The can contains BPA.

Progresso Rich & Hearty Lentil and Andouille Sausage
(1 cup)
210 calories
11 g fat (3.5 g saturated)
670 mg sodium
22 g carbohydrates
4 g fiber
10 g protein

With tons of nitrites and chemicals listed in the ingredients, this soup is a major don't.

Campbell's Homestyle Healthy Request Chicken with Whole Grain Pasta
(1 cup)
100 calories
2 g fat (0.5 g saturated)
410 mg sodium
13 g carbohydrates
1 g fiber
7 g protein

Where's the fiber?

Swanson 100% Natural Vegetable Broth
(1 cup)
10 calories
0 g fat (0 g saturated)
800 mg sodium
2 g carbohydrates
0 g fiber
0 g protein

Sure, this has fewer calories than Kitchen Basics, but it packs almost four times the sodium! Just. Say. No.

Campbell's Slow Kettle Style Soup Tomato & Sweet Basil Bisque
(1 cup)
260 calories
16 g fat (10 g saturated)
790 mg sodium
33 g carbohydrates
2 g fiber
4 g protein

This soup contains as much sugar as 66 Chocolate Teddy Graham cookies.

Bars

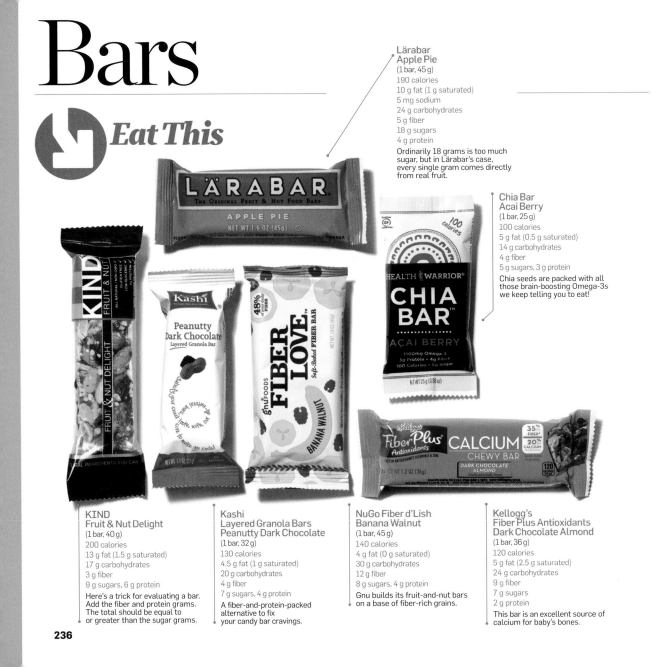

Eat This

Lärabar Apple Pie
(1 bar, 45 g)
190 calories
10 g fat (1 g saturated)
5 mg sodium
24 g carbohydrates
5 g fiber
18 g sugars
4 g protein

Ordinarily 18 grams is too much sugar, but in Lärabar's case, every single gram comes directly from real fruit.

Chia Bar Acai Berry
(1 bar, 25 g)
100 calories
5 g fat (0.5 g saturated)
14 g carbohydrates
4 g fiber
5 g sugars, 3 g protein

Chia seeds are packed with all those brain-boosting Omega-3s we keep telling you to eat!

KIND Fruit & Nut Delight
(1 bar, 40 g)
200 calories
13 g fat (1.5 g saturated)
17 g carbohydrates
3 g fiber
9 g sugars, 6 g protein

Here's a trick for evaluating a bar. Add the fiber and protein grams. The total should be equal to or greater than the sugar grams.

Kashi Layered Granola Bars Peanutty Dark Chocolate
(1 bar, 32 g)
130 calories
4.5 g fat (1 g saturated)
20 g carbohydrates
4 g fiber
7 g sugars, 4 g protein

A fiber-and-protein-packed alternative to fix your candy bar cravings.

NuGo Fiber d'Lish Banana Walnut
(1 bar, 45 g)
140 calories
4 g fat (0 g saturated)
30 g carbohydrates
12 g fiber
8 g sugars, 4 g protein

Gnu builds its fruit-and-nut bars on a base of fiber-rich grains.

Kellogg's Fiber Plus Antioxidants Dark Chocolate Almond
(1 bar, 36 g)
120 calories
5 g fat (2.5 g saturated)
24 g carbohydrates
9 g fiber
7 g sugars
2 g protein

This bar is an excellent source of calcium for baby's bones.

Quaker
Oatmeal to Go
Apples with Cinnamon
(1 bar, 60 g)

220 calories
4 g fat (1 g saturated)
44 g carbohydrates
5 g fiber
22 g sugars, 4 g protein

There's far more sugar, brown sugar, and high-fructose corn syrup than apple.

PowerBar
Vanilla Crisp
(1 bar, 57 g)

240 calories
3.5 g fat (0.5 g saturated)
45 g carbohydrates
1 g fiber
26 g sugars
8 g protein

Four kinds of sugar make this "performance" bar sweeter than a Kit Kat.

Savor It Try a less sweet option like Kind's Honey Smoked BBQ.

Three-Peat
Pump up your Omega-3s with an Oatmega bar—they're full of 'em.

Not That!

Nature's Path
Organic Choconut
(1 bar, 35 g)

140 calories
4.5 g fat (1.5 g saturated)
24 g carbohydrates
2 g fiber
11 g sugars
2 g protein

Sugar, in its various guises, appears five times in this ingredient statement.

Odwalla Bar
Banana Nut
(1 bar, 56 g)

220 calories
5 g fat (0.5 g saturated)
39 g carbohydrates
5 g fiber
17 g sugars, 4 g protein

Don't be duped by "brown rice syrup," the first ingredient in this bar. It's a euphemism for sugar.

PowerBar Triple Threat
Caramel Peanut Fusion
(1 bar, 45 g)

200 calories
9 g fat (4 g saturated)
23 g carbohydrates
3 g fiber
12 g sugars
12 g protein

This "Power" bar is just caramel and "chocolate coating."

Nature Valley
Crunchy Oats 'n Honey (
(2 bars, 42 g)

190 calories
7 g fat (1 g saturated)
29 g carbohydrates
2 g fiber
11 g sugars, 3 g protein

This bar has twice as much sugar as it does fiber and protein combined. That makes it a great example of the sort of snack you want to avoid.

Crackers

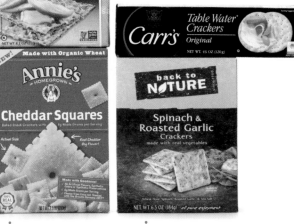

Carr's Table Water Crackers
(4 crackers, 14 g)
60 calories
1 g fat (0 g saturated)
80 mg sodium
10 g carbohydrates
<1 g fiber

White crackers don't have much nutritional value, it's true, but plain crackers are a lifesaver for many women suffering from morning sickness—and these have half the fat of Keebler Club crackers.

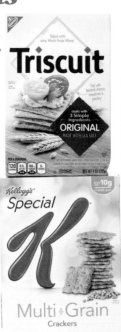

![Eat This]

Nabisco Triscuit Baked Whole Grain Wheat Original
(6 crackers, 28 g)
120 calories
2.5 g fat (0.5 g saturated)
160 mg sodium
20 g carbohydrates
3 g fiber

You can't beat the purity of this recipe: whole wheat, oil, and salt. Period.

Wasa Crispbread Fiber
(2 crispbreads, 20 g)
60 calories
1 g fat (0 g saturated)
90 mg sodium
14 g carbohydrates
5 g fiber

The wheat germ, bran, and whole grain rye in these crackers really amp up the fiber content here.

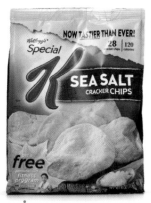

Kellogg's Special K Sea Salt Cracker Chips
(28 crackers, 30 g)
120 calories
4 g fat (0 g saturated)
220 mg sodium
21 g carbohydrates
3 g fiber

Potato starch is used to bolster this cracker chip's fiber content.

Special K Multi-Grain Crackers
(24 crackers, 30 g)
120 calories
3 g fat (0 g saturated)
170 mg sodium
23 g carbohydrates
3 g fiber

This is as few calories as you can reasonably expect in a serving of whole-grain crackers.

Annie's Cheddar Squares
(27 pieces, 30 g)
150 calories
7 g fat (0.5 g saturated)
250 mg sodium
19 g carbohydrates
1 g fiber

A touch of fiber and real cheese save this cracker.

Back to Nature Spinach & Roasted Garlic Crackers
(20 crackers, 30 g)
130 calories
4 g fat (0 g saturated)
190 mg sodium
22 g carbohydrates
2 g fiber

The first two ingredients here are unbleached wheat flour and whole grain wheat flour. Plus, there's actually dried spinach in here, which helps boost your iron levels.

Keebler Club Crackers,
Original
(13 pieces, 30 g)
130 calories
4 g fat (0.5 g saturated)
230 mg sodium
22 g carbohydrates
3 g fiber
Definitely plain, but not so great.

Nabisco Ritz Bits
Sandwiches Cheese
(13 pieces, 31 g)
160 calories
9 g fat (3 g saturated)
160 mg sodium
18 g carbohydrates
0 g fiber
Soiled with sugar and partially
hydrogenated cottonseed oil.

*When suffering morning sickness,
try a few plain, low-fat crackers, like the Carr's on the left.
Eat two and call me in the morning.*

Not That!

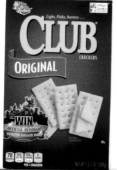
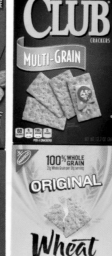
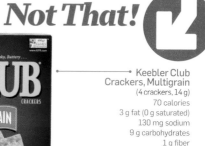

Keebler Club
Crackers, Multigrain
(4 crackers, 14 g)
70 calories
3 g fat (0 g saturated)
130 mg sodium
9 g carbohydrates
1 g fiber
If you're looking for a plain
cracker to calm your tummy,
you can find one with
a lot less fat than this!

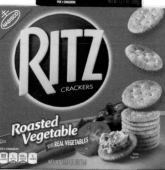
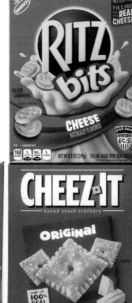
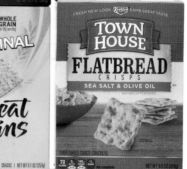

Ritz Roasted Vegetable
(5 crackers, 16 g)
80 calories
3 g fat (1 g saturated)
150 mg sodium
10 g carbohydrates
0 g fiber

As the name suggests, this box
contains a handful of dehydrated
vegetables. The problem is, the main
ingredient is still refined flour, and
it's bogged down with hydrogenated
oils and high-fructose corn syrup.

Sunshine
Cheez-It Original
(27 crackers, 30 g)
150 calories
8 g fat (2 g saturated)
230 mg sodium
17 g carbohydrates
<1 g fiber

Cheez-Its' lack of fiber
prevents these crackers from
having a meaningful impact
on hunger. If you're
going to snack, do so smartly.

Nabisco
Wheat Thins Original
(16 crackers, 31 g)
140 calories
5 g fat (1 g saturated)
230 mg sodium
22 g carbohydrates
3 g fiber

Wheat Thins rely heavily on
refined grains, which means less
protein and fiber in each serving.

Keebler Town House
Flatbread Crisps
Sea Salt & Olive Oil
(16 crackers, 30 g)
140 calories
4 g fat (0 g saturated)
280 mg sodium
22 g carbohydrates
<1 g fiber

The 4 grams of fat here come
from soybean oil.

239

Chips

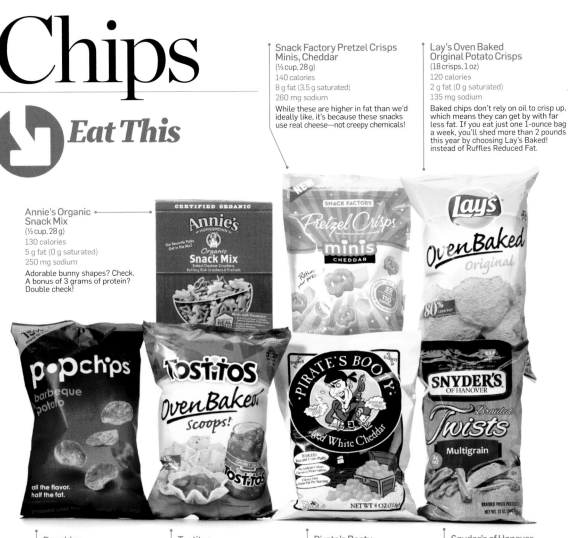

Eat This

Snack Factory Pretzel Crisps Minis, Cheddar
(⅓ cup, 28 g)
140 calories
8 g fat (3.5 g saturated)
260 mg sodium

While these are higher in fat than we'd ideally like, it's because these snacks use real cheese—not creepy chemicals!

Lay's Oven Baked Original Potato Crisps
(18 crisps, 1 oz)
120 calories
2 g fat (0 g saturated)
135 mg sodium

Baked chips don't rely on oil to crisp up, which means they can get by with far less fat. If you eat just one 1-ounce bag a week, you'll shed more than 2 pounds this year by choosing Lay's Baked! instead of Ruffles Reduced Fat.

Annie's Organic Snack Mix
(½ cup, 28 g)
130 calories
5 g fat (0 g saturated)
250 mg sodium

Adorable bunny shapes? Check. A bonus of 3 grams of protein? Double check!

Popchips Barbeque Potato
(20 chips, 1 oz)
120 calories
4 g fat (0 g saturated)
200 mg sodium

More crunch than a baked chip, yet less fat than a fried chip.

Tostitos Oven Baked Scoops!
(16 chips, 1 oz)
120 calories
3 g fat (0.5 g saturated)
140 mg sodium

This is the healthiest salsa-shoveling device on the shelf.

Pirate's Booty Aged White Cheddar
(1 ounce, 28 g)
130 calories
5 g fat (1 g saturated)
140 mg sodium

The cheesey snack you already love is pretty low in sodium and even has 2 g of protein per serving.

Snyder's of Hanover Braided Twists Multigrain
(8 twists, 30 g)
120 calories
2 g fat (0 g saturated)
160 mg sodium

The 3 grams of fiber in each serving make this a respectable snack.

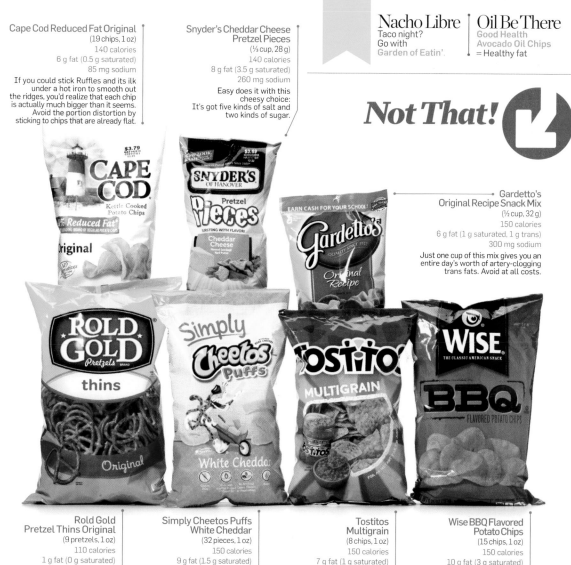

Cape Cod Reduced Fat Original
(19 chips, 1 oz)
140 calories
6 g fat (0.5 g saturated)
85 mg sodium

If you could stick Ruffles and its ilk under a hot iron to smooth out the ridges, you'd realize that each chip is actually much bigger than it seems. Avoid the portion distortion by sticking to chips that are already flat.

Snyder's Cheddar Cheese Pretzel Pieces
(⅓ cup, 28 g)
140 calories
8 g fat (3.5 g saturated)
260 mg sodium

Easy does it with this cheesy choice: It's got five kinds of salt and two kinds of sugar.

Nacho Libre
Taco night?
Go with
Garden of Eatin'.

Oil Be There
Good Health
Avocado Oil Chips
= Healthy fat

Not That!

Gardetto's Original Recipe Snack Mix
(½ cup, 32 g)
150 calories
6 g fat (1 g saturated, 1 g trans)
300 mg sodium

Just one cup of this mix gives you an entire day's worth of artery-clogging trans fats. Avoid at all costs.

Rold Gold Pretzel Thins Original
(9 pretzels, 1 oz)
110 calories
1 g fat (0 g saturated)
490 mg sodium

More sodium than a large order of McDonald's fries.

Simply Cheetos Puffs White Cheddar
(32 pieces, 1 oz)
150 calories
9 g fat (1.5 g saturated)
290 mg sodium

Being "puffed" doesn't cut down on fat, calories, or sodium.

Tostitos Multigrain
(8 chips, 1 oz)
150 calories
7 g fat (1 g saturated)
110 mg sodium

The "multiple" grains in this bag consist almost entirely of corn.

Wise BBQ Flavored Potato Chips
(15 chips, 1 oz)
150 calories
10 g fat (3 g saturated)
210 mg sodium

This bag contains a bunch of processing junk like monosodium glutamate and artificial colors.

Dips & Spreads

Wholly Guacamole Guaca Salsa
(2 tbsp, 30 g)
35 calories
3 g fat (0 g saturated)
110 mg sodium

Avocados are the first of only seven ingredients, all of which you likely keep stocked in your kitchen.

Desert Pepper Black Bean Dip Spicy
(2 tbsp, 33 g)
25 calories
0 g fat
240 mg sodium

This jar contains a trio of nutritional A-listers: black beans, tomatoes, and green bell peppers.

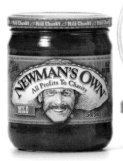
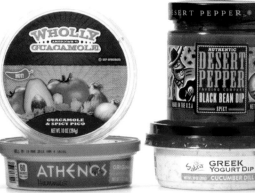
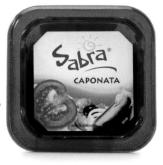

Newman's Own Mild Salsa
(2 tbsp, 32 g)
10 calories
0 g fat
65 mg sodium

We balked when Ronald Reagan tried to turn ketchup into a vegetable, but if someone did the same for salsa, a legitimate nutritional superpower, we'd throw our support behind it.

Athenos Hummus Original
(2 tbsp, 28 g)
60 calories
3.5 g fat (0 g saturated)
170 mg sodium

Made with real olive oil, which lends an authentic flavor and more heart-healthy fats.

Sabra Greek Yogurt Dip in Cucumber Dill
(2 tbsp, 30 g)
40 calories
2.5 g fat (1.5 g saturated)
95 mg sodium

All the benefits of filling Greek yogurt, with a refreshing taste of cukes.

Sabra Caponata
(2 tbsp, 28 g)
30 calories
2.5 g fat (0 g saturated)
140 mg sodium

Built from potent Mediterranean produce like eggplants and tomatoes, this dip is perfect for dressing up chicken or fish or spreading on a pita.

My favorite spread is hummus. Little more than chickpeas, olive oil, sesame seeds, and sometimes garlic make it your go-to condiment. Smear it on sandwiches or set it out as a hunger-quashing dip with vegetables or crackers.

Not That!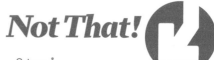

Frito's Bean Dip, Original
(2 tbsp, 33 g)
35 calories
1 g fat (0 g saturated)
190 mg sodium

This party starter is a non-starter: it's made with corn maltodextrin, a caloric sweetener.

Ortega Guacamole Style Dip
(2 tbsp (31 g)
45 calories
3 g fat (0 g saturated fat)
190 mg sodium

This stuff is basically just water, canola oil, and corn starch with less than 2 percent "avocado powder." Yuck.

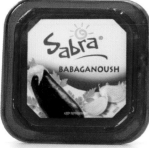
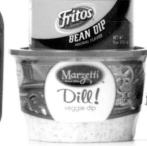
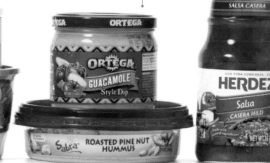

Sabra Babaganoush
(2 tbsp, 28 g)
70 calories
7 g fat (1 g saturated)
180 mg sodium

Babaganoush traditionally gets its creaminess from tahini and roasted eggplant, but Sabra cheats by loading its version with mayonnaise.

Marzetti Dill Veggie Dip
(2 tbsp, 30 g)
110 calories
12 g fat (3 g saturated)
180 mg sodium

This dip is mostly sour cream. The veggies you see on the package? You'll have to supply those yourself.

Sabra Roasted Pine Nut Hummus
(2 tbsp, 28 g)
80 calories
6 g fat (1 g saturated)
130 mg sodium

Instead of the traditional olive oil, Sabra's ingredient statement lists "soybean and/or canola oil."

Herdez Salsa Casera Mild
(2 tbsp, 31 g)
10 calories
0 g fat
270 mg sodium

Be on the watch for elevated sodium in salsa. Combined with some salty chips, you could easily approach half a day's sodium intake.

243

Dressings

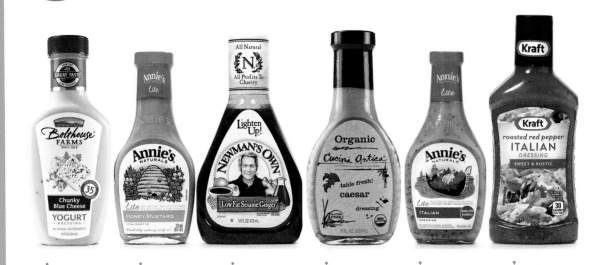

**Bolthouse Farms
Yogurt Dressing
Chunky Blue
Cheese**
(2 tbsp, 30 g)
35 calories
2.5 g fat (1 g saturated)
135 mg sodium

Bolthouse Farms casts
yogurt as the star in
classic flavors such as
ranch, honey mustard,
Thousand Island, and
blue cheese, allowing
you to swap out
vegetable oil for worth-
while hits of calcium
and probiotic bacteria.

**Annie's Naturals
Lite Honey Mustard
Vinaigrette**
(2 tbsp, 31 g)
40 calories
3 g fat (0 g saturated)
125 mg sodium

After water, mustard
is the main ingredient,
a surprising rarity
among honey mustard
dressings.

**Newman's Own
Lite Low Fat
Sesame Ginger**
(2 tbsp, 30 g)
35 calories
1.5 g fat (0 g saturated)
330 mg sodium

Oil is just a supporting
role in this zingy
dressing that contains
tummy-soothing ginger.

**Cucina Antica
Organic Caesar
Dressing**
(2 tbsp, 30 g)
50 calories
5 g fat (1 g saturated)
300 mg sodium

A touch of Romano
cheese, not an
excess of cheap oil,
supplies rich flavor for
a fraction of the fat.

**Annie's
Italian Lite**
(2 tbsp, 30 g)
25 calories
1.5 g fat (0 g saturated)
120 mg sodium

No preservatives,
no high-fructose corn
syrup, and totally
vegan? This one can
perfectly top any salad!

**Kraft
Roasted Red
Pepper Italian
with Parmesan**
(2 tbsp, 32 g)
40 calories
2 g fat (0 g saturated)
340 mg sodium

The bulk of this bottle
is filled with vinegar
and tomato puree,
a huge improvement
over the typical
oil-based formula.

BEST DRESSED
Look for a dressing that has less than 50 calories per serving, and less than 5 grams of fat.

POUR CHOICES
The best brands have vinegar, ginger, soy or other natural ingredients coming before "oil."

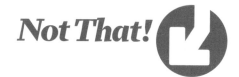

Not That!

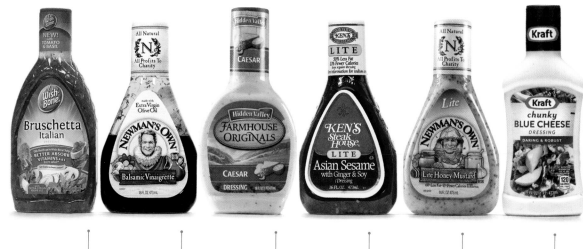

Wish-Bone Bruschetta Italian
(2 tbsp, 30 ml)
60 calories
5 g fat (1 g saturated)
340 mg sodium

The front label boasts about olive oil, but the ingredient statement reveals that it accounts for less than 2 percent of the recipe.

Newman's Own Balsamic Vinaigrette
(2 tbsp, 30 g)
90 calories
9 g fat (1 g saturated)
280 mg sodium

Save cash and calories by making your own vinaigrette at home: Mix two parts olive oil with one part balsamic, plus salt and pepper.

Hidden Valley Farmhouse Originals Caesar
(2 tbsp, 30 ml)
120 calories
11 g fat
(1.5 g saturated)
220 mg sodium

Hidden in this valley, you'll find MSG and propylene glycol, an ingredient also found in anti-freeze. We don't remember those from any farm.

Ken's Steak House Lite Asian Sesame with Ginger and Soy
(2 tbsp, 30 g)
70 calories
4 g fat
(0.5 g saturated)
390 mg sodium

After water, sugar is the first ingredient in this bottle, which is why each serving packs 7 grams of the sweet stuff.

Newman's Own Lite Honey Mustard Dressing
(2 tbsp, 30 g)
70 calories
4 g fat
(0.5 g saturated)
240 mg sodium

Keep in mind that "lite" is a relative term.

Kraft Chunky Blue Cheese Dressing
2 tbsp, 29 g
120 calories
12 g fat (2 g saturated)
310 mg sodium

Virtually every calorie in this bottle comes from soybean oil, which doesn't contain the same heart-healthy elements as olive or canola oil. Even the leanest of salads would end up a fatty mess with this drizzled on top!

Cookies

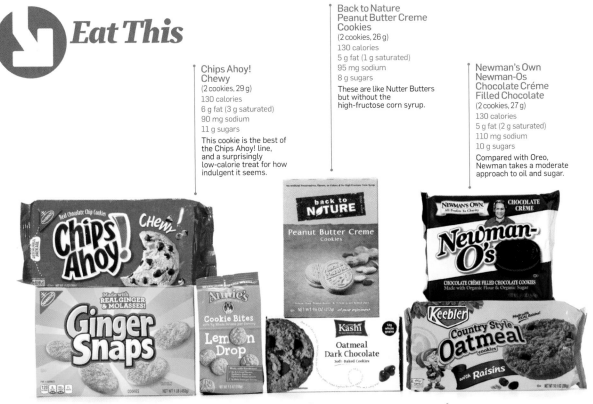

Eat This

Chips Ahoy! Chewy
(2 cookies, 29 g)
130 calories
6 g fat (3 g saturated)
90 mg sodium
11 g sugars

This cookie is the best of the Chips Ahoy! line, and a surprisingly low-calorie treat for how indulgent it seems.

Back to Nature Peanut Butter Creme Cookies
(2 cookies, 26 g)
130 calories
5 g fat (1 g saturated)
95 mg sodium
8 g sugars

These are like Nutter Butters but without the high-fructose corn syrup.

Newman's Own Newman-Os Chocolate Créme Filled Chocolate
(2 cookies, 27 g)
130 calories
5 g fat (2 g saturated)
110 mg sodium
10 g sugars

Compared with Oreo, Newman takes a moderate approach to oil and sugar.

Nabisco Ginger Snaps
(4 cookies, 28 g)
120 calories
2.5 g fat (0 g saturated)
190 mg sodium
11 g sugars

Eating a handful of small cookies instead of one regular cookie is a good strategy—it can help you feel like you're eating more than you actually are.

Annie's Lemon Drop Cookie Bites
(7 cookies, 30 g)
140 calories
7 g fat (2.5 g saturated)
60 mg sodium
7 g sugars

I love these because they "drop" the high-fructose corn syrup and artificial colors—and taste delicious.

Kashi Oatmeal Dark Chocolate Soft-Baked Cookies
(1 cookie, 30 g)
130 calories
5 g fat (1 g saturated)
65 mg sodium
8 g sugars

Thanks to oats, rye, barley, and buckwheat, Kashi's cookie has more fiber (4 grams) than a standard slice of whole-wheat bread.

Keebler Country Style Oatmeal with Raisins
(2 cookies, 28 g)
140 calories
6 g fat (2 g saturated)
100 mg sodium
8 g sugars

Raisins will always trump chocolate chips or candy pieces as a cookie mix-in.

Choco-Not! *When you get a cookie craving, enjoy a few, but not the whole box. A study from the University of Adelaide found that moms who eat a ton of junk food birth babies addicted to sugar and fat.*

Not That!

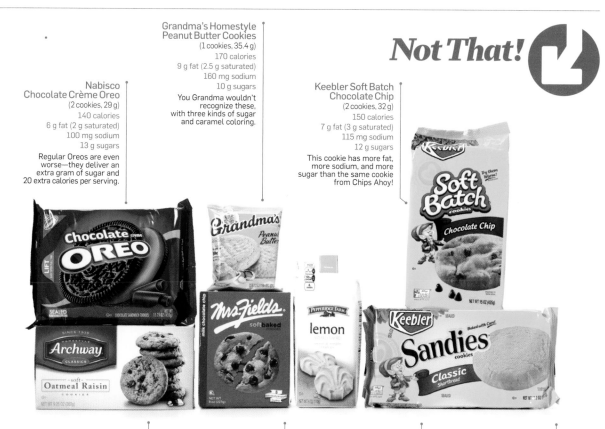

Grandma's Homestyle Peanut Butter Cookies
(1 cookies, 35.4 g)
170 calories
9 g fat (2.5 g saturated)
160 mg sodium
10 g sugars

You Grandma wouldn't recognize these, with three kinds of sugar and caramel coloring.

Nabisco Chocolate Crème Oreo
(2 cookies, 29 g)
140 calories
6 g fat (2 g saturated)
100 mg sodium
13 g sugars

Regular Oreos are even worse—they deliver an extra gram of sugar and 20 extra calories per serving.

Keebler Soft Batch Chocolate Chip
(2 cookies, 32 g)
150 calories
7 g fat (3 g saturated)
115 mg sodium
12 g sugars

This cookie has more fat, more sodium, and more sugar than the same cookie from Chips Ahoy!

Archway Classics Soft Oatmeal Raisin
(1 cookies, 33 g)
140 calories
4.5 g fat (2 g saturated)
85 mg sodium
12 g sugars

Add just one of these 140-calorie cookies to your daily diet and you'll gain nearly 15 pounds this year.

Mrs. Fields Milk Chocolate Chip
(1 cookie, 28 g)
130 calories
6 g fat (3 g saturated)
110 mg sodium
11 g sugars

The dearth of fiber ensures that this will pass straight through your belly, spike your blood sugar, and convert quickly to flab.

Pepperidge Farm Lemon Cookies
(4 cookies, 32 g)
160 calories
8 g fat (3 g saturated)
105 mg sodium
8 g sugars

Just a bit too high in saturated fat.

Keebler Sandies Simply Shortbread
(2 cookies, 31 g)
160 calories
9 g fat (4 g saturated)
90 mg sodium
7 g sugars

We love the low sugar count, but not the heavy deposits of soybean and palm oils.

247

Candy

Eat This

Nestlé 100 Grand
(1 package, 43 g)
190 calories
8 g fat (5 g saturated)
22 g sugars

This is an Eat This, Not That! Hall of Famer, routinely beating out more common chocolate bars by 80 or more calories.

Hershey's Kit Kat
(1 package, 42 g)
210 calories
11 g fat (7 g saturated)
21 g sugars

The wafer core is light and porous, which saves you calories over the denser bars.

Jelly Belly Mini Pack
(9 beans, 10 g)
35 calories
0 g fat
7 g sugars

At 4 calories each bean, they're the slimmest way to enjoy cotton candy and toasted marshmallows.

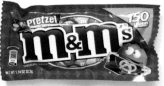

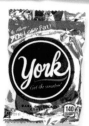

Pretzel M&M's
(1 bag, 32 g)
150 calories
4.5 g fat (3 g saturated)
17 g sugars

The original milk chocolate core has been replaced with pretzel, which is low in calories by confectionary standards. As a result, you trade in a boatload of sugar for a satisfying crunch.

York Peppermint Pattie
(1 patty, 39 g)
140 calories
2.5 g fat (1.5 g saturated)
25 g sugars

For a smaller treat, go with York Miniatures. You can have three for about the same number of calories.

Hershey's Take 5
(1 package, 42 g)
210 calories
11 g fat (5 g saturated)
18 g sugars

The pretzel core saves you a boatload of calories.

Green & Black's 85%
(12 pieces, 40 g)
250 calories
20 g fat (12 g saturated)
8 g sugars

This bar is particularly smooth for the high cacao content. This dark chocolate can increase serotonin and endorphin levels in the brain, reducing stress and elevating mood.

Justin's Dark Chocolate Mini Peanut Butter Cups
(3.5 pieces, 40 g)
210 calories
14 g fat (7 g saturated)
17 g sugars

Justin's is devoted to sustainable, organic ingredients, and their candies are made with ingredients you can pronounce.

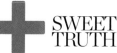

SWEET TRUTH

Anything that's labeled "made with chocolate," "chocolaty," or "chocolate-coated" likely doesn't contain very much—if any—cocoa butter, the ingredient responsible for dark chocolate's waist-whittling effect.

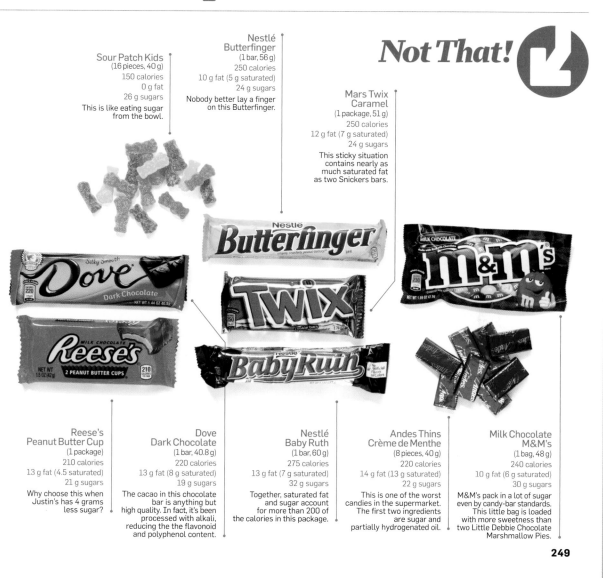

Sour Patch Kids
(16 pieces, 40 g)
150 calories
0 g fat
26 g sugars
This is like eating sugar from the bowl.

Nestlé Butterfinger
(1 bar, 56 g)
250 calories
10 g fat (5 g saturated)
24 g sugars
Nobody better lay a finger on this Butterfinger.

Not That!

Mars Twix Caramel
(1 package, 51 g)
250 calories
12 g fat (7 g saturated)
24 g sugars
This sticky situation contains nearly as much saturated fat as two Snickers bars.

Reese's Peanut Butter Cup
(1 package)
210 calories
13 g fat (4.5 saturated)
21 g sugars
Why choose this when Justin's has 4 grams less sugar?

Dove Dark Chocolate
(1 bar, 40.8 g)
220 calories
13 g fat (8 g saturated)
19 g sugars
The cacao in this chocolate bar is anything but high quality. In fact, it's been processed with alkali, reducing the the flavonoid and polyphenol content.

Nestlé Baby Ruth
(1 bar, 60 g)
275 calories
13 g fat (7 g saturated)
32 g sugars
Together, saturated fat and sugar account for more than 200 of the calories in this package.

Andes Thins Crème de Menthe
(8 pieces, 40 g)
220 calories
14 g fat (13 g saturated)
22 g sugars
This is one of the worst candies in the supermarket. The first two ingredients are sugar and partially hydrogenated oil.

Milk Chocolate M&M's
(1 bag, 48 g)
240 calories
10 g fat (6 g saturated)
30 g sugars
M&M's pack in a lot of sugar even by candy-bar standards. This little bag is loaded with more sweetness than two Little Debbie Chocolate Marshmallow Pies.

249

Frozen Breakfast

Eat This

Jimmy Dean Delights Turkey Sausage Breakfast Bowl (1 bowl, 198 g)

240 calories
8 g fat (3.5 g saturated)
720 mg sodium
1 g sugars
2 g fiber
22 g protein

Protein accounts for 40 percent of the calories, which increases your odds of making it to lunch without a Snickers.

Special K Flatbread Breakfast Sandwich, Egg, Vegetables & Pepper Jack Cheese (1 sandwich, 95 g)

150 calories
7 g fat (3 g saturated)
430 mg sodium
5 g fiber
3 g sugars
10 g protein

Best part about this sandwich? Despite what the box says below, it's now got a new recipe that's 30 calories less.

Amy's Black Beans & Tomatoes Breakfast Burrito (1 burrito, 170 g)

270 calories
8 g fat (1 g saturated)
540 mg sodium
3 g sugars
6 g fiber
12 g protein

Black beans are one of the healthiest foods on the planet.

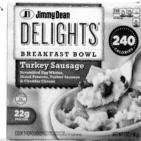

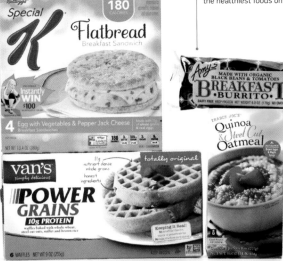

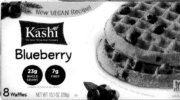

Kashi Blueberry Waffles (2 waffles, 72 g)

140 calories
5 g fat (0.5 g saturated)
310 mg sodium
3 g sugars
7 g fiber
3 g protein

Blueberries figure prominently in these first-rate waffles, explaining the huge hit of fiber.

Van's Power Grains (2 waffles, 85 g)

210 calories
7 g fat (0.5 g saturated)
180 mg sodium
3 g fiber
6 g sugars
10 g protein

Packed with cracked red wheat, steel cut oats, millet, and brown rice.

Trader Joe's Frozen Qunioa and Steelcut Oatmeal (1 serving, 227 g)

180 calories
2 g fat (0 g saturated)
50 mg sodium
9 g sugars
5 g protein

Steel cut oats are higher in fiber and have a lower glycemic index than regular oatmeal.

Entrées

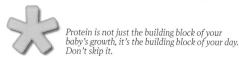

Protein is not just the building block of your baby's growth, it's the building block of your day. Don't skip it.

Bob Evans'
Sausage, Egg & Cheese Burrito
(68 g)
350 calories
21 g fat (6 g saturated)
810 mg sodium
0 g sugars
1 g fiber
13 g protein

This has twice the fat as
the Jimmy Dean bowl.

Kellogg's Special K
Flatbread Breakfast Sandwich
Sausage Egg & Cheese
(1 sandwich, 116 g)
220 calories
12 g fat (4 g saturated)
700 mg sodium
3 g sugars
5 g fiber
14 g protein

The ingredients list is a novel.

Not That!

Lean Pockets Sausage,
Egg & Cheese (1 piece, 127 g)
270 calories
8 g fat (4 g saturated)
370 mg sodium
5 g sugars
0 g fiber
29 g protein

More than 150 of these calories are
carbohydrates, which is not
how you want to start your day.

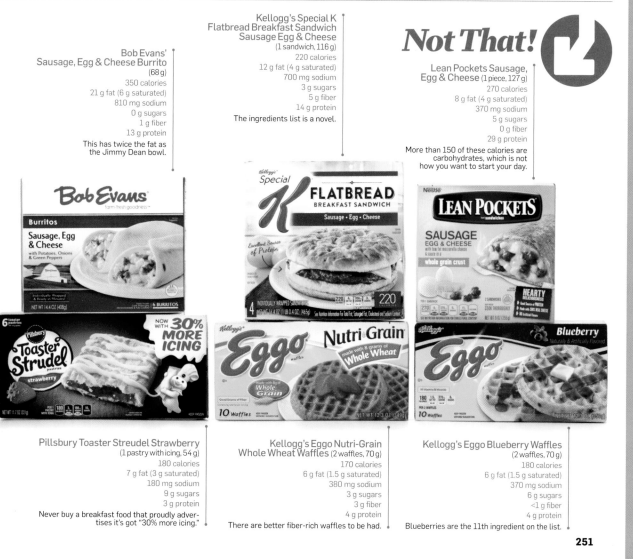

Pillsbury Toaster Streudel Strawberry
(1 pastry with icing, 54 g)
180 calories
7 g fat (3 g saturated)
180 mg sodium
9 g sugars
3 g protein

Never buy a breakfast food that proudly adver-
tises it's got "30% more icing."

Kellogg's Eggo Nutri-Grain
Whole Wheat Waffles (2 waffles, 70 g)
170 calories
6 g fat (1.5 g saturated)
380 mg sodium
3 g sugars
3 g fiber
4 g protein

There are better fiber-rich waffles to be had.

Kellogg's Eggo Blueberry Waffles
(2 waffles, 70 g)
180 calories
6 g fat (1.5 g saturated)
370 mg sodium
6 g sugars
<1 g fiber
4 g protein

Blueberries are the 11th ingredient on the list.

251

Frozen Pizzas

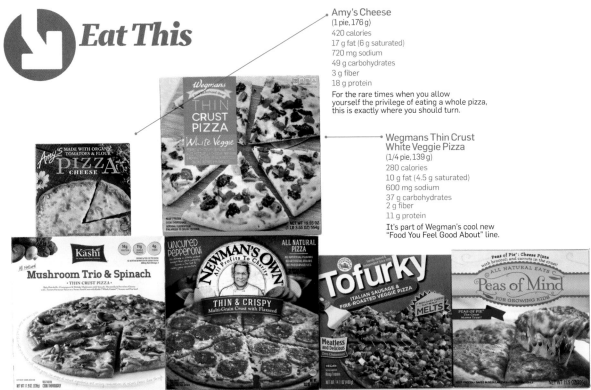

Eat This

Amy's Cheese
(1 pie, 176 g)
420 calories
17 g fat (6 g saturated)
720 mg sodium
49 g carbohydrates
3 g fiber
18 g protein

For the rare times when you allow yourself the privilege of eating a whole pizza, this is exactly where you should turn.

Wegmans Thin Crust White Veggie Pizza
(1/4 pie, 139 g)
280 calories
10 g fat (4.5 g saturated)
600 mg sodium
37 g carbohydrates
2 g fiber
11 g protein

It's part of Wegman's cool new "Food You Feel Good About" line.

Kashi Stone-Fired Thin Crust Pizza Mushroom Trio & Spinach
(⅓ pie, 113 g)
250 calories
9 g fat (4.5 g saturated)
660 mg sodium
28 g carbohydrates
4 g fiber
14 g protein

This pie features more pesto than cheese, a healthy swap.

Newman's Own Thin & Crispy Uncured Pepperoni
(⅓ pie, 125 g)
320 calories
16 g fat (6 g saturated)
800 mg sodium
31 g carbohydrates
2 g fiber
15 g protein

The rare instance in which pepperoni is OK, because this brand skips the nitrates.

Tofurky Italian Sausage & Fire Roasted Veggie
(⅓ pie, 132 g)
270 calories
6 g fat (1 g saturated)
320 mg sodium
40 g carbohydrates
5 g fiber
13 g protein

Tofurky's lactose-free "cheese" is made using protein, flour, and oils.

Peas of Mind Cheese
(⅓ pie, 109 g)
240 calories
5 g fat (2 g saturated)
510 mg sodium
36 g carbohydrates
2 g fiber
11 g protein

They snuck broccoli and carrots into the crust. Clever devils!

SLICE THE FAT

Aim for a serving that's less than 320 calories, with fewer than 6 grams of saturated fat. Many pizzas have double that!

LIVE AND LET PIE

Try Vitalicious— it's only five inches in diameter and goes light on the cheese.

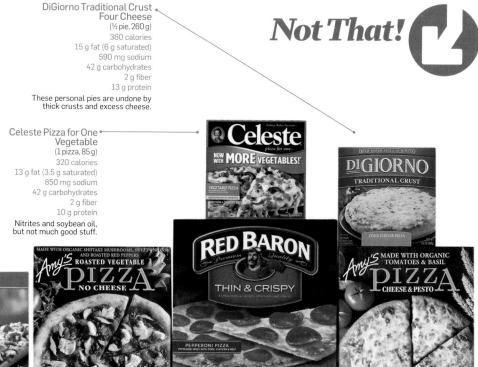

Not That!

DiGiorno Traditional Crust Four Cheese
(½ pie, 260 g)
360 calories
15 g fat (6 g saturated)
590 mg sodium
42 g carbohydrates
2 g fiber
13 g protein

These personal pies are undone by thick crusts and excess cheese.

Celeste Pizza for One Vegetable
(1 pizza, 85 g)
320 calories
13 g fat (3.5 g saturated)
850 mg sodium
42 g carbohydrates
2 g fiber
10 g protein

Nitrites and soybean oil, but not much good stuff.

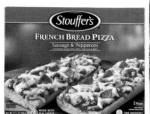

Stouffer's French Bread Sausage & Pepperoni
(2 pieces, 177 g)
460 calories
24 g fat (8 g saturated)
880 mg sodium
43 g carbohydrates
4 g fiber
17 g protein

One contains the saturated fat of 16 Burger King Chicken Tenders.

Amy's Roasted Vegetable No Cheese
(⅓ pie, 113 g)
280 calories
9 g fat (1.5 g saturated)
540 mg sodium
42 g carbohydrates
3 g fiber
7 g protein

For the lactose intolerant, there are options closer to the real thing.

Red Baron Thin & Crispy Pepperoni Pizza
(⅓ pie, 139 g)
360 calories
16 g fat (8 g saturated)
840 mg sodium
40 g carbohydrates
2 g fiber
14 g protein

Even the Baron's thin-crust pies pack too much of the bad stuff.

Amy's Whole Wheat Crust Cheese & Pesto
(⅓ pie, 132 g)
360 calories
18 g fat (4 g saturated)
680 mg sodium
37 g carbohydrates
4 g fiber
13 g protein

The crust is the least nutritious part of any pie, and unfortunately, Amy's is just a little bit too thick.

253

Frozen Pasta Ent

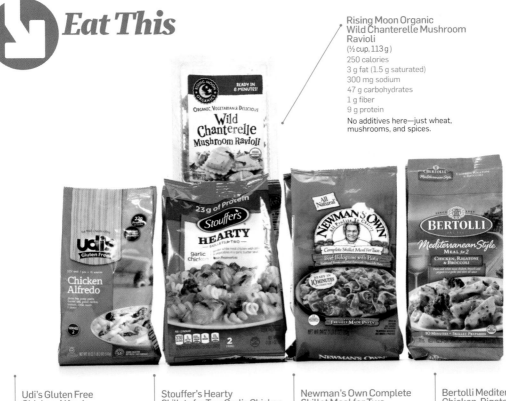

Eat This

Rising Moon Organic Wild Chanterelle Mushroom Ravioli
(½ cup, 113 g)
250 calories
3 g fat (1.5 g saturated)
300 mg sodium
47 g carbohydrates
1 g fiber
9 g protein

No additives here—just wheat, mushrooms, and spices.

Udi's Gluten Free Chicken Alfredo
(½ bag, 255 g)
400 calories
20 g fat (11 g saturated)
690 mg sodium
36 g carbohydrates
2 g fiber
22 g protein

If you're sensitive to gluten, I recommend this light and springy pasta, made with rice flour.

Stouffer's Hearty Skillets for Two Garlic Chicken
(½ bag, 326 g)
330 calories
5 g fat (0 g saturated)
870 mg sodium
48 g carbohydrates
5 g fiber
23 g protein

You get a big bang of protein for very, very little fat. And if you already have a family, it's a quick way to feed them, too.

Newman's Own Complete Skillet Meal for Two Beef Bolognese
(½ package, 340 g)
390 calories
11 g fat (3.5 g saturated)
920 mg sodium
44 g carbohydrates
4 g fiber
24 g protein

This'll satisfy your Chef Boyardee cravings but has half the salt.

Bertolli Mediterranean Style Chicken, Rigatoni & Broccoli
(½ package, 340 g)
400 calories
16 g fat (4 g saturated)
860 mg sodium
44 g carbohydrates
4 g fiber
20 g protein

You're worried about saving for her college fund. He's worried he'll get fat. Bring back the romance with this dinner for two.

rées

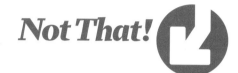

Not That!

Stouffer's Cheese Ravioli with Meat Sauce
(1 entrée, 251 g)
310 calories
12 g fat (6 g saturated)
1,030 mg sodium
36 g carbohydrates
3 g fiber
14 g protein

This has 160 mg more sodium and 9 g less protein than the Stouffer's dish on the left.

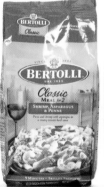

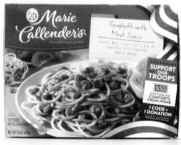

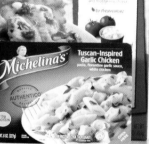

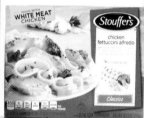

Bertolli Classic Shrimp Scampi & Linguine
(½ package, 340 g)
480 calories
20 g fat (9 g saturated)
980 mg sodium
56 g carbohydrates
3 g fiber
18 g protein

Romano takes a heavy-handed approach with cream, as demonstrated by the exorbitant glut of saturated fat in this dish.

Marie Callender's Spaghetti with Meat Sauce
(1 meal, 425 g)
530 calories
15 g fat (4.5 g saturated)
1,000 mg sodium
76 g carbohydrates
7 g fiber
22 g protein

This is as good as the past you'd find at a Marie Callender's restaurant. Unfortunately, it's also as caloric.

Michelina's Tuscan Inspired Garlic Chicken
(1 package, 227 g)
290 calories
7 g fat (3.5 g saturated)
580 mg sodium
43 g carbohydrates
2 g fiber
14 g protein

Given all the ingredients—including salt, sugars, and artificial flavors—you'd think this would have more protein.

Stouffer's Chicken Fettuccini Alfredo
(1 package, 297 g)
570 calories
27 g fat (7 g saturated)
850 mg sodium
55 g carbohydrates
5 g fiber
26 g protein

Alfredo sauce contains any of the following: oil, butter, cheese, cream, and egg yolk. In other words, it's a full-fat assault.

255

Frozen Fish Entr

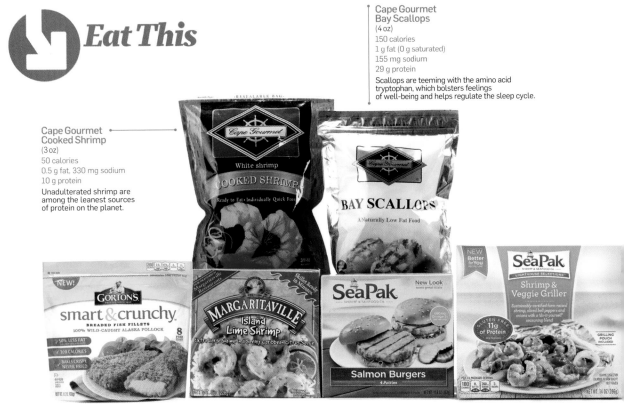

Eat This

**Cape Gourmet
Bay Scallops**
(4 oz)
150 calories
1 g fat (0 g saturated)
155 mg sodium
29 g protein
Scallops are teeming with the amino acid tryptophan, which bolsters feelings of well-being and helps regulate the sleep cycle.

**Cape Gourmet
Cooked Shrimp**
(3 oz)
50 calories
0.5 g fat, 330 mg sodium
10 g protein
Unadulterated shrimp are among the leanest sources of protein on the planet.

**Gortons's
Smart & Crunchy Breaded
Fish Fillets**
(2 fillets, 108 g)
200 calories
6 g fat (2.5 g saturated)
470 mg sodium
11 g protein
Half the fat, lower cal, more protein than Van de Kamp's—plus no potentially sketchy plastic tray.

**Margaritaville Island
Lime Shrimp**
(6 shrimp, 4 oz)
240 calories
11 g fat (3 g saturated)
330 mg sodium
12 g protein
These shrimp have also been tossed in butter. The difference is quantity; here it's a light bath, but in SeaPak's scampi it's a tidal wave.

SeaPak Salmon Burgers
(1 burger, 91 g)
110 calories
5 g fat (1 g saturated)
340 mg sodium
16 g protein
Toss this on the grill, then sandwich it between a toasted bun with arugula, grilled onions, and Greek yogurt spiked with olive oil, garlic, and fresh dill.

**Gourmet
Shrimp & Veggie Griller**
(⅓ package, 132 g)
100 calories
1 g fat (0 g saturated)
300 mg sodium
11 g protein
American interpretations of Asian cuisine tend to be high in sodium, but this solid blend of fiber and protein more than makes up for it.

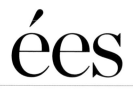

ées

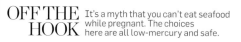

OFF THE
HOOK — It's a myth that you can't eat seafood while pregnant. The choices here are all low-mercury and safe.

Mrs. Paul's Fried Scallops
(13 scallops)
260 calories
11 g fat (4 g saturated)
700 mg sodium
12 g protein

Scallops are among the sea's greatest gifts to man. Spoiling them with the fryer treatment is an abomination. You end up with more calories from fat than protein.

Not That!

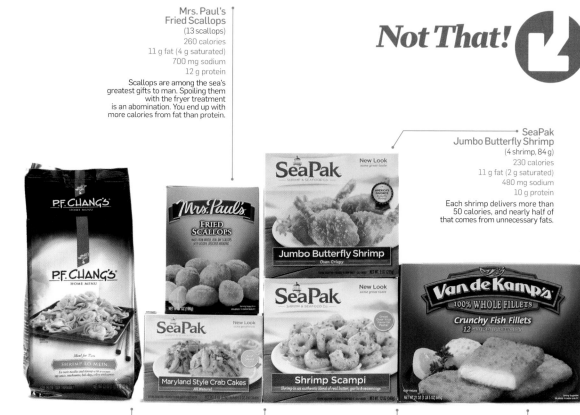

SeaPak Jumbo Butterfly Shrimp
(4 shrimp, 84 g)
230 calories
11 g fat (2 g saturated)
480 mg sodium
10 g protein

Each shrimp delivers more than 50 calories, and nearly half of that comes from unnecessary fats.

P.F. Chang's Home Menu Shrimp Lo Mein
(½ package, 312 g)
390 calories
12 g fat (1.5 g saturated)
740 mg sodium
16 g protein

Chang's sauce is polluted with three kinds of oil.

SeaPak Maryland Style Crab Cakes
(1 crab cake with 1 oz sauce, 113 g)
240 calories
13 g fat (1.5 g saturated)
830 mg sodium
11 g protein

These crab cakes deliver more starchy filler than actual shellfish. Somewhere, a Marylander is shaking his head.

SeaPak Shrimp Scampi
(6 shrimp, 113 g)
340 calories
31 g fat (12 g saturated)
480 mg sodium
12 g protein

Shrimp are essentially pure protein, so it's puzzling to find that protein accounts for just 13 percent of this entrée's calories.

Van de Kamp's Crunchy Fish Fillets
(2 fillets, 110 g)
210 calories
10 g fat (3.5 g saturated)
690 mg sodium
9 g protein

You know what makes the breading crunchy? The same thing that makes it 150 percent more caloric and 267 percent fattier: oil.

Frozen Chicken

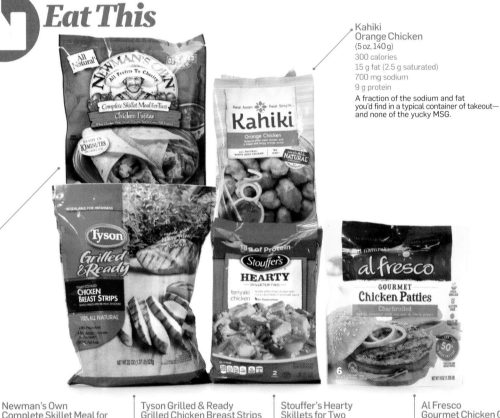

Eat This

**Kahiki
Orange Chicken**
(5 oz, 140 g)
300 calories
15 g fat (2.5 g saturated)
700 mg sodium
9 g protein

A fraction of the sodium and fat
you'd find in a typical container of takeout—
and none of the yucky MSG.

**Newman's Own
Complete Skillet Meal for
Two Chicken Fajitas**
(½ package)
310 calories
6 g fat (0.5 g saturated)
660 mg sodium
21 g protein

Keep yourself and baby
healthy with this
vitamin C-packed protein fiesta.

**Tyson Grilled & Ready
Grilled Chicken Breast Strips**
(3 oz, 84 g)
100 calories
2.5 g fat (0.5 g saturated)
420 mg sodium
19 g protein

Less fat and more protein than
a nugget, and just as easy to make.

**Stouffer's Hearty
Skillets for Two
Teriyaki Chicken**
(½ package, 354 g)
320 calories
3 g fat (1 g saturated)
740 mg sodium
18 g protein

Intense hunger and savory cravings
are no match for this hearty—
yet low cal—meal solution.

**Al Fresco
Gourmet Chicken Grillers
Lightly Seasoned**
(1 patty, 98 g)
150 calories
8 g fat (2 g saturated)
340 mg sodium
15 g protein

Flavored with lemon peel and spices,
this patty has a homemade flavor.

Entrées

Bang for Your Buck Chicken McNuggets have 33 ingredients. Banquet Chicken Breast Patties have 32. For cleaner eating, choose the Tyson.

Not That!

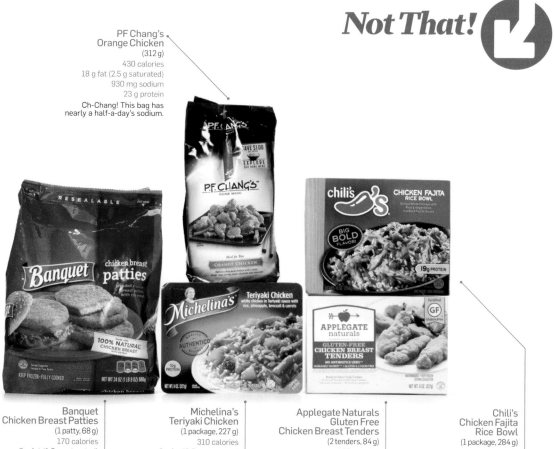

PF Chang's Orange Chicken
(312 g)
430 calories
18 g fat (2.5 g saturated)
930 mg sodium
23 g protein
Ch-Chang! This bag has nearly a half-a-day's sodium.

Banquet Chicken Breast Patties
(1 patty, 68 g)
170 calories
9 g fat (1.5 g saturated)
300 mg sodium
8 g protein
Banquet's breading adds excess calories and zero value. It also gets demerits for using BHT, a potentially dangerous preservative.

Michelina's Teriyaki Chicken
(1 package, 227 g)
310 calories
3 g fat (0.5 g saturated)
830 mg sodium
10 g protein
This zappable dish may save you some time, but it serves up more sodium and less protein than its stovetop rival.

Applegate Naturals Gluten Free Chicken Breast Tenders
(2 tenders, 84 g)
130 calories
5 g fat (0.5 g saturated)
360 mg sodium
11 g protein
"Gluten-free" may distract you from the fact that these nuggets get their extra calories from carbs.

Chili's Chicken Fajita Rice Bowl
(1 package, 284 g)
370 calories
10 g fat (3.5 g saturated)
960 mg sodium
20 g protein
Made with more rice than chicken, there's nothing fun about this party in a bowl.

259

Frozen Sides, Sna

Eat This

Health is Wealth
Spring Rolls, Vegetable
(2 rolls, 45 g)
70 calories
2 g fat (0 g saturated)
290 mg sodium
12 g carbohydrates
By simply ditching the fatty cheese and bacon, these savory vegan spring rolls beat the competition by a long stretch.

Alexia Sweet Potato Puffs
(84 g)
140 calories
4.5 g fat (tk g saturated)
230 mg sodium
23 g carbohydrates
A dusting of vinegar, mustard seed, turmeric, and paprika give these tater-tot-esque bites flavor.

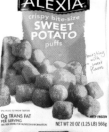

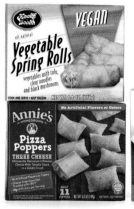

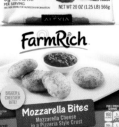

Annie's Three Cheese Pizza Poppers (6 pieces, 81 g)
180 calories
5 g fat (2 g saturated)
300 mg sodium
27 g carbohydrates
These bite-sized snacks are filled with cheesy goodness—yet manage to stay light in the fat and sodium department.

Farm Rich Mozzarella Bites
(4 pieces, 45 g)
160 calories
7 g fat (3 g saturated)
280 mg sodium
16 g carbohydrates
For something that's 90% bread and cheese the fat and carb count isn't too out of control.

Ore-Ida Steak Fries
(7 fries, 84 g)
110 calories
3 g fat (0.5 g saturated)
290 mg sodium
19 g carbohydrates
A serving of these hulking spuds contains fewer than half the calories you'd find in the average medium order of fast-food fries.

Cascadian Farm Shoe String French Fries
(3 oz, 85 g)
110 calories
5 g fat (1 g saturated)
10 mg sodium
17 g carbohydrates
Cascadian Farm tosses these fries in apple juice, the sugar from which caramelizes into a crisp, golden crust.

cks & Appetizers

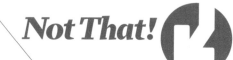
Not That!

**T.G.I. Friday's
Chicken Quesadilla Rolls**
(2 pieces, 83 g)
230 calories
10 g fat (3 g saturated, 1 g trans)
470 mg sodium
27 g carbohydrates
9 g protein

Frozen flour tortillas are little
trans-fat delivery systems.

Ore-Ida Tater Tots
(86 g)
160 calories
8 g fat (1.5 g saturated)
420 mg sodium
20 g carbohydrates

You're not in middle school anymore.
Eat Ore-Ida's Steak Fries instead.

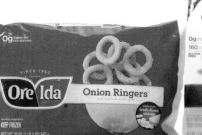
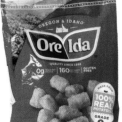
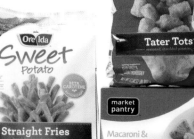

**Ore-Ida
Onion Ringers**
(3 pieces, 81 g)
180 calories
10 g fat (2 g saturated)
160 mg sodium
21 g carbohydrates

Each ring harbors more than
3 grams of fat. Fries are
almost always the better choice.

**Ore-Ida
Sweet Potato Straight Fries**
(22 fries, 84 g)
160 calories
8 g fat (0.5 g saturated)
160 mg sodium
21 g carbohydrates

A raw sweet potato has more fiber
and vitamin A than a raw russet
potato. But this one's filled with fat.

**Market Pantry
Mac & Cheese Bites**
(4 pieces, 90 g)
240 calories
12 g fat (5 g saturated)
660 mg sodium
26 g carbohydrates

If cheese is what you crave,
there are far less fatty and
starchy ways to get your fix.

Totino's Pizza Rolls Cheese
(6 rolls, 85 g)
220 calories
9 g fat (2.5 g saturated)
410 mg sodium
26 g carbohydrates

Aside from its poor nutritionals,
these rolls are coated with
titanium dioxide, a whitening agent
your liver doesn't need.

Ice Creams

Eat This

Breyers
Black Raspberry Chocolate
(½ cup, 67 g)
140 calories
4 g fat (3 g saturated)
16 g sugars

The secret to a low-calorie ice cream is simple: Lead off with something lighter than cream. This one uses regular milk first and cream last.

Häagen-Dazs
Chocolate Sorbet
(½ cup, 105 g)
130 calories
0.5 g fat (0 g saturated)
21 g sugars

One of the few Häagen-Dazs products that we can actually stand behind.

Edy's Rich & Creamy
Grand Coffee
(½ cup, 65 g)
140 calories
7 g fat (4 g saturated)
14 g sugars

Careful—it's made with real coffee, so it's not the best choice right before bed.

Turkey Hill Light Recipe
Moose Tracks
(½ cup, 61 g)
140 calories
6 g fat (2.5 g saturated)
15 g sugars

Swirled ice cream flecked with chocolate peanut butter cups—you won't find a more decadent dessert with fewer calories.

Edy's Slow Churned
Mint Chocolate Chip
(½ cup, 60 g)
120 calories
4.5 g fat (3 g saturated)
13 g sugars

Edy's Slow Churned line leans more heavily on milk than cream, which keeps the calories in check.

So Delicious
Chocolate Velvet
(½ cup, 81 g)
130 calories
3.5 g fat (0.5 g saturated)
14 g sugars

So Delicious cuts the fat without needing to make up for it with an extra hit of sugar.

Breyers Natural
Vanilla
(½ cup, 66 g)
130 calories
7 g fat (4 g saturated)
14 g sugars

Breyers Natural has earned our allegiance for both its low-calorie concoctions and the simplicity of its ingredient statements.

WE ALL SCREAM FOR...

Breyers! Their Original line keeps the calorie count reasonable, with only a few all-natural ingredients.

THE HOT SCOOP

The best ice cream is just milk, sugar, cream and maybe a little bit of fruit.

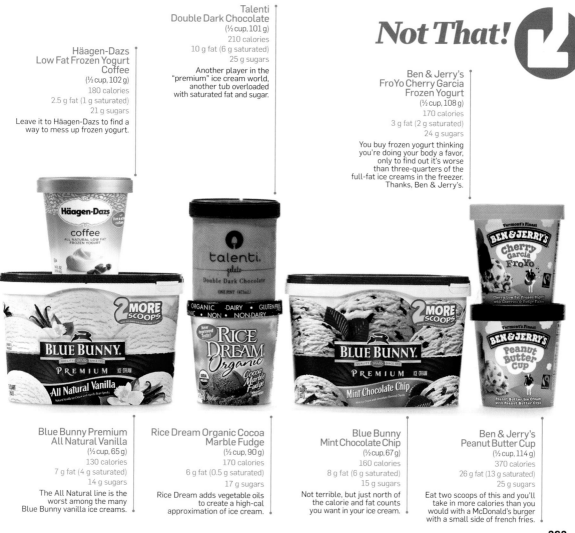

Talenti Double Dark Chocolate
(½ cup, 101 g)

210 calories

10 g fat (6 g saturated)

25 g sugars

Another player in the "premium" ice cream world, another tub overloaded with saturated fat and sugar.

Häagen-Dazs Low Fat Frozen Yogurt Coffee
(½ cup, 102 g)

180 calories

2.5 g fat (1 g saturated)

21 g sugars

Leave it to Häagen-Dazs to find a way to mess up frozen yogurt.

Not That!

Ben & Jerry's FroYo Cherry Garcia Frozen Yogurt
(½ cup, 108 g)

170 calories

3 g fat (2 g saturated)

24 g sugars

You buy frozen yogurt thinking you're doing your body a favor, only to find out it's worse than three-quarters of the full-fat ice creams in the freezer. Thanks, Ben & Jerry's.

Blue Bunny Premium All Natural Vanilla
(½ cup, 65 g)

130 calories

7 g fat (4 g saturated)

14 g sugars

The All Natural line is the worst among the many Blue Bunny vanilla ice creams.

Rice Dream Organic Cocoa Marble Fudge
(½ cup, 90 g)

170 calories

6 g fat (0.5 g saturated)

17 g sugars

Rice Dream adds vegetable oils to create a high-cal approximation of ice cream.

Blue Bunny Mint Chocolate Chip
(½ cup, 67 g)

160 calories

8 g fat (6 g saturated)

15 g sugars

Not terrible, but just north of the calorie and fat counts you want in your ice cream.

Ben & Jerry's Peanut Butter Cup
(½ cup, 114 g)

370 calories

26 g fat (13 g saturated)

25 g sugars

Eat two scoops of this and you'll take in more calories than you would with a McDonald's burger with a small side of french fries.

Frozen Treats

Eat This

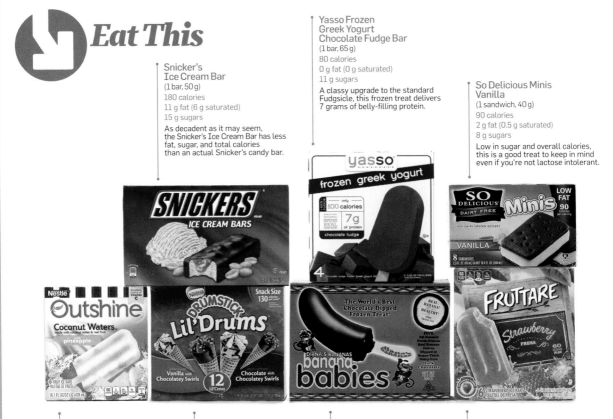

Snicker's Ice Cream Bar
(1 bar, 50 g)
180 calories
11 g fat (6 g saturated)
15 g sugars

As decadent as it may seem, the Snicker's Ice Cream Bar has less fat, sugar, and total calories than an actual Snicker's candy bar.

Yasso Frozen Greek Yogurt Chocolate Fudge Bar
(1 bar, 65 g)
80 calories
0 g fat (0 g saturated)
11 g sugars

A classy upgrade to the standard Fudgsicle, this frozen treat delivers 7 grams of belly-filling protein.

So Delicious Minis Vanilla
(1 sandwich, 40 g)
90 calories
2 g fat (0.5 g saturated)
8 g sugars

Low in sugar and overall calories, this is a good treat to keep in mind even if you're not lactose intolerant.

Nestlé Outshine Coconut Waters with Pineapple
(1 bar, 60 grams)
60 calories
0 g fat (0 g saturated)
14 g sugars

Escape to coco-mo.

Nestlé Drumstick Lil' Drums Vanilla with Chocolatey Swirls
(1 cone, 43 g)
110 calories
5 g fat (3.5 g saturated)
10 g sugars

The perfect portion for an after-dinner indulgence.

Diana's Bananas Banana Babies Dark Chocolate
(1 piece, 60 g)
130 calories
6 g fat (3.5 g saturated)
14 g sugars

Banana, chocolate, and peanut oil. You don't find a frozen treat with a simpler recipe.

Fruttare Strawberry
(1 bar, 56 g)
60 calories
0 g fat (0 g saturated)
0 mg sodium
11 g sugars

Still sugary, but at least has some real fruit!

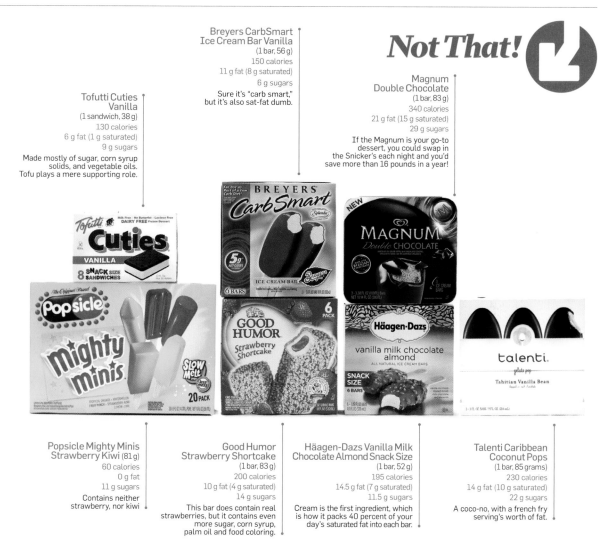

Breyers CarbSmart Ice Cream Bar Vanilla
(1 bar, 56 g)
150 calories
11 g fat (8 g saturated)
6 g sugars
Sure it's "carb smart," but it's also sat-fat dumb.

Not That!

Magnum Double Chocolate
(1 bar, 83 g)
340 calories
21 g fat (15 g saturated)
29 g sugars
If the Magnum is your go-to dessert, you could swap in the Snicker's each night and you'd save more than 16 pounds in a year!

Tofutti Cuties Vanilla
(1 sandwich, 38 g)
130 calories
6 g fat (1 g saturated)
9 g sugars
Made mostly of sugar, corn syrup solids, and vegetable oils. Tofu plays a mere supporting role.

Popsicle Mighty Minis Strawberry Kiwi (81 g)
60 calories
0 g fat
11 g sugars
Contains neither strawberry, nor kiwi

Good Humor Strawberry Shortcake
(1 bar, 83 g)
200 calories
10 g fat (4 g saturated)
14 g sugars
This bar does contain real strawberries, but it contains even more sugar, corn syrup, palm oil and food coloring.

Häagen-Dazs Vanilla Milk Chocolate Almond Snack Size
(1 bar, 52 g)
195 calories
14.5 g fat (7 g saturated)
11.5 g sugars
Cream is the first ingredient, which is how it packs 40 percent of your day's saturated fat into each bar.

Talenti Caribbean Coconut Pops
(1 bar, 85 grams)
230 calories
14 g fat (10 g saturated)
22 g sugars
A coco-no, with a french fry serving's worth of fat.

Juices

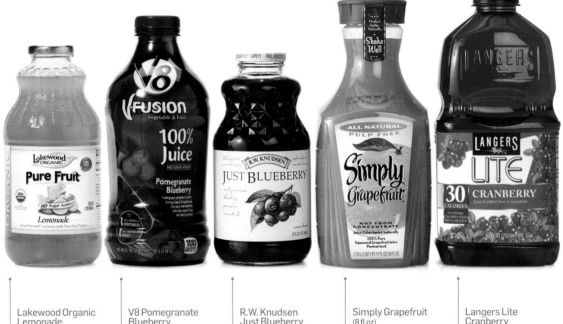

Eat This

Lakewood Organic Lemonade
(8 fl oz)
100 calories
0 g fat
23 g sugars
This drink is sweetened with grape juice instead of sugar.

V8 Pomegranate Blueberry
(8 fl oz)
100 calories
0 g fat
22 g sugars
You get a full serving of vegetables and fruits in one new blend.

R.W. Knudsen Just Blueberry
(8 fl oz)
100 calories
0 g fat
19 g sugars
Blueberries are bursting with brain-boosting antioxidants, and R.W. Knudsen's juice is the only one to give you 100 percent blueberries.

Simply Grapefruit
(8 fl oz)
100 calories
0 g fat
25 g sugars
Grapefruit is the most underrated juice in the cooler. It's delicious, it's naturally low in sugar, and it delivers a dose of cancer-fighting lycopene.

Langers Lite Cranberry
(8 fl oz)
30 calories
0 g fat
8 g sugars
Cranberries make for a tart juice, which is why you routinely see 15 or more grams of sugar added to each serving. Langers Lite keeps it simple.

Not That!

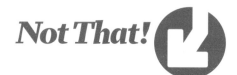

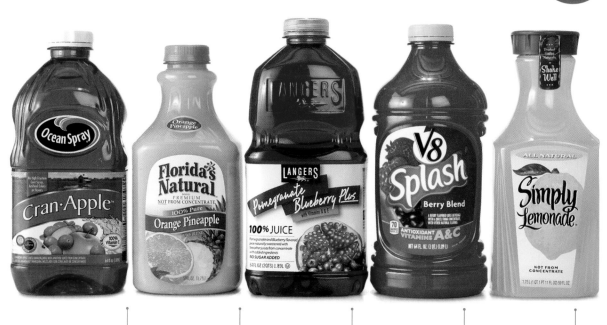

Ocean Spray Cran-Apple
(8 fl oz)

120 calories
0 g fat
31 g sugars

This bottle, like so many in Ocean Spray's lineup, contains only 15 percent juice. Water and sugar are the first two ingredients.

Florida's Natural 100% Pure Orange Pineapple
(8 fl oz)

130 calories
0 g fat
30 g sugars

It's hard to find fault with 100-percent juice products, but blends like this tend to pack in too much sugar.

Langers Pomegranate Blueberry Plus
(8 fl oz)

130 calories
0 g fat
30 g sugars

There's more sugar in this bottle than there are blueberries or pomegranates.

V8 Splash Berry Blend
(8 fl oz)

70 calories
0 g fat
16 g sugars

Splash is unfit to carry the V8 brand name. It's made with artificial colors, high-fructose corn syrup, and a pathetic 5 percent juice.

Simply Lemonade
(8 fl oz)

120 calories
0 g fat
28 g sugars

Contains only 11 percent juice. The rest of the bottle is pure sugar water. Most lemonades follow the same disappointing formula.

267

Chapter

8

Cook This, Not That!

A Trimester-by-Trimester Breakdown

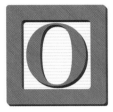

ONE DAY, YEARS FROM NOW, the little baby in your belly will be cooking you mother's day breakfast in bed. And if you're lucky, it might even be edible.

Until then, the best gift you can give them—every day—is a home-cooked meal. The team at *Fit Pregnancy* know this better than anyone. The online magazine for moms-to-be has been a tremendous resource for healthy eating since 1993. In this chapter, you'll find a cornucopia of their best recipes—complete meals for every trimester that focus on the vitamins and minerals you and your baby really need.

The first trimester is abundant in lower-calorie dishes that comprise a lot of citrus and nutrients shown to help reduce the risk of neural defects and other early-pregnancy issues. The meals for the second trimester are slightly higher in calories per serv-ing. For the third trimester, you'll find slightly higher-calorie dishes and food that will store (and even freeze) well for after the baby comes.

Finally, we've included a few beverages that don't contain alcohol but are so festive you won't miss it.

Cooking at home is essential for your child's health—but also for yours, if you're worried about weight gain. Imagine that, over the course of a week, you cooked pizza, burgers, steak, waffles and other staples at home, instead of going out to eat them. You'd save a whopping 3,385 calories just in that seven days—essentially a pound's worth of flab. That's 50 pounds in just 1 year. So go ahead: Ciao down Bella! At home, when you can.

Weeks 0–14

- Breakfast
- Lunch
- Dinner
- Dessert

First Trimester

Your first trimester is when you want to provide the building blocks for a healthy baby. Folate, vitamin C, omega-3s, and protein are crucial now, but you don't need to gain a bunch of weight just yet. So these recipes are light, but mighty. Enjoy.

California Barley Bowl with Lemony Yogurt Sauce

Folate-rich avocados and protein-packed almonds both boost your baby's development. The lemony yogurt sauce also helps quell queasiness.

PREP • Active: 10 minutes • Total: 10 minutes • Serves 2

Almonds	Avocado	Barley	Yogurt	Lemon
healthy fat and omega-3 oils for brain development	vitamins E, K, C, B6, and B5, potassium, folate and dietary fiber	high in fiber to keep your blood pressure low and promote good digestion	good source of calcium for your and baby's bones and teeth	calms morning sickness; vitamin C is essential for tissue repair, bone growth and repair, and healthy skin

INGREDIENTS

1½ cups cooked barley, warmed

¼ cup sliced almonds, toasted

¼ teaspoon kosher salt

1 small ripe avocado, peeled, pitted and sliced

Lemony Yogurt Sauce (below)

Flaky sea salt (such as Maldon)

Freshly ground black pepper

Lemony Yogurt Sauce:

½ cup plain yogurt

1 teaspoon grated lemon zest

1 teaspoon freshly squeezed lemon juice

1 tablespoon chopped fresh chives

Pinch of kosher salt

DIRECTIONS

- In a small bowl, stir the barley, almonds, and kosher salt together.
- Scoop into 2 individual bowls and top with avocado and a few generous spoonfuls of yogurt sauce. Sprinkle with flaky salt and pepper.

LEMONY YOGURT SAUCE DIRECTIONS

- Whisk all ingredients together in a small bowl. Refrigerate any leftover sauce.

Per Serving: 183 calories, 4 g protein, 32g carbohydrates, 7g fat (1g sat), 73 mg calcium, 2 mg iron, 14 mcg folate, 7 g fiber, 247 mg sodium

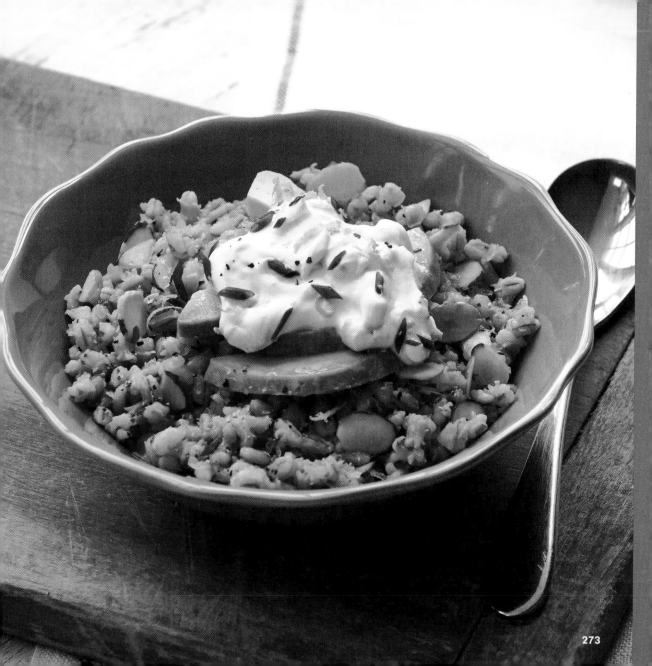

Blackberry–Bran Muffins

This easy, vegan grab-and-go muffin morsel keeps your system running smoothly with a hefty dose of fiber; the flaxseed also is packed with omega-3 oils.

PREP • Active: 25 minutes • Total: 75 minutes • Makes 12 servings

Bran & Oats	Flaxseed	Lemon juice	Almond milk
fiber to keep you regular	vegan source of omega-3 oils for baby brain development	morning sickness fighter, vitamin C for baby cell development and immunity	vegan source of protein for muscle growth and calcium for bones and teeth

INGREDIENTS

- 1 **cup plain, unsweetened almond milk**
- 1 **tablespoon fresh lemon juice**
- 2 **cups wheat bran**
- ½ **cup old-fashioned rolled oats**
- 1 **tablespoon ground flaxseed**
- ¼ **cup hot water** (about 180 F)
- ¾ **cup packed light brown sugar**
- ½ **cup unsweetened applesauce**
- ¼ **cup canola oil**
- 1¼ **cups whole-wheat pastry flour**
- 1 **teaspoon baking powder**
- 1 **teaspoon baking soda**
- ½ **teaspoon ground cinnamon**
- ½ **teaspoon sea salt**
- 1 **cup fresh blackberries**

DIRECTIONS

- Position a rack in the lower third of the oven and preheat to 350 F. Lightly oil 12 muffin cups or use paper liners.

- In a large mixing bowl, whisk together almond milk and lemon juice. Let stand for 5 to 10 minutes to thicken into "buttermilk." Whisk again and stir in the bran and oats.

- In a medium mixing bowl, combine flaxseed with hot water. Allow to sit for 5 to 10 minutes until it thickens. Whisk the brown sugar, applesauce and oil into flaxseed mixture. Add this mixture to the bowl with the "buttermilk" combo, stirring until batter is combined.

- In another medium mixing bowl, whisk together the flour, baking powder, baking soda, cinnamon, and salt. Add this mixture to the batter, stirring just until combined. Do not overmix. Fold in the berries.

- Fill each muffin cup with a heaping ½ cup of butter. The muffin cups should be full and the muffins rounded at the top, with blackberries in each.

- Bake for 35 to 40 minutes, or until muffins are firm to the touch and a toothpick inserted comes out clean.

- Let cool in the tin for 10 minutes. Turn out muffins and continue to cool them on a wire rack for another 10 minutes before serving.

Per Serving (1 muffin): 183 calories, 4 g protein, 32 g carbohydrates, 7 g fat (1g sat.), 73 mg calcium, 2 mg iron, 14 mcg folate, 7 g fiber, 247 mg sodium

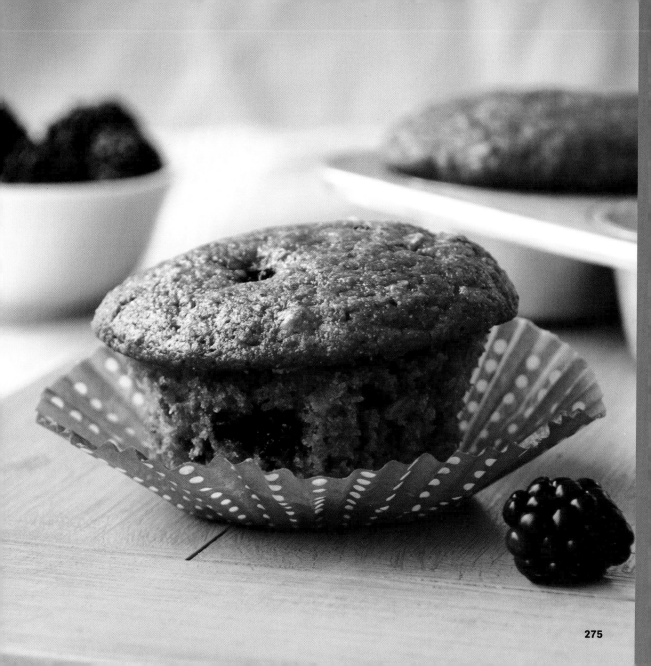

Cranberry-Orange Buttermilk Scones

These quick and easy baked goods not only satisfy a sweet craving, but also deliver a hit of citrus (a boon for alleviating morning sickness) and cranberries (which guard against UTIs, something you're prone to during pregnancy).

PREP ● Active: 20 minutes ● Total: 30 minutes ● Makes 12

Cranberries
can prevent and treat mild UTIs

Oranges
source of vitamin C for your and baby's immunity, eases morning sickness

INGREDIENTS

- 2 **cups all-purpose flour**
- ¼ **cup plus 2 tablespoons sugar**
- 2 **teaspoons baking powder**
- 1 **teaspoon baking soda**
- ¼ **teaspoon salt**
- ⅔ **cup dried cranberries**
- ⅔ **cup plus 2 tablespoons low-fat buttermilk**
- ¼ **cup canola oil**
- 1 **teaspoon grated orange zest**
- 1 **large egg**

DIRECTIONS

- Preheat oven to 400 F

- In a large bowl, combine flour, ¼ cup sugar, baking powder, baking soda, and salt; stir in cranberries

- In another bowl, whisk 2/3 cup buttermilk, oil, zest, and egg. Pour into flour mixture, stirring until combined.

- Turn out onto floured surface; knead five or six times. Flatten to 9-inch round. With a 2-inch wide glass, cut out 6 scones. Combine scraps and repeat. Place on baking sheet and sprinkle with remaining sugar and buttermilk.

- Bake 10 minutes until golden brown. Let cool on wire rack just until warm.

Per Serving (1 scone): 174 calories, 3 g protein, 28 g carbohydrates, 6 g fat (1g sat.), 80 mg calcium, 1mg iron, 41 mcg folate, 1 g fiber, 250 mg sodium

Crispy Thai Slaw with Curry Dressing

Instead of spooning out a mayo-heavy and calorie-laden packaged slaw, try this easy, spicy-sour Asian version. A cornucopia of crunchy vegetables provides fiber to keep things moving and the dense nutrition you and your baby need now.

PREP ● Active: 15 minutes ● Total: 15 minutes ● Makes 6 servings

Ginger	Curry powder	Peanuts	Vegetables
Helps ease morning sickness and indigestion, aids in absorption of nutrients	Contains turmeric, a great natural anti-inflammatory	Healthy fats and plant protein for cell development	Green, leafy vegetables are high in folate to protect against birth defects

INGREDIENTS

- 4 **cups shredded Napa or green cabbage**
- 2 **medium carrots, sliced into matchsticks**
- 1 **red bell pepper**
- 3 **scallions (white and green parts), trimmed and sliced**
- ¼ **cup light coconut milk**
- 1 **tablespoon grated or finely minced ginger**
- 1 **tablespoon fish sauce**
- 1 **tablespoon rice vinegar**
- 2 **teaspoons curry powder**
- 2 **teaspoons sesame oil**
- ⅓ **cup cilantro, chopped**
- ⅓ **cup roasted unsalted peanuts, chopped**
- **Lime wedges**

DIRECTIONS

- In a large bowl, toss together cabbage, carrots, red bell pepper and scallion. In a small bowl, whisk together coconut milk, ginger, fish sauce, vinegar, curry powder, and sesame oil. Toss dressing with vegetables.

- Divide slaw among serving plates and garnish with cilantro and peanuts. Serve with lime wedges.

Per Serving: 115 calories, 4 g protein, 11g carbohydrates, 7g fat (2g sat.), 42 mg calcium, 1 mg iron, 70 mcg folate, 4 g fiber, 329 mg sodium

Salmon Burgers with Avocado Sauce

There's nothing fishy about swapping out traditional beef patties for ones made with omega-3 packed salmon. Studies show that this nutritional powerhouse may decrease the risk of pre- and postnatal depression. Plus, slathering on the punchy avocado sauce adds a dose of folate, a B-vitamin that protects against birth defects.

PREP ● Active: 25 minutes ● Total: 30 minutes ● Makes 4 servings

Avocado	Salmon	Sour cream	Whole grain bun
folate to prevent neural tube defects	omega-3 oils for baby's brain and to prevent pre- and postnatal depression	a dollop of calcium for baby's (and your) bones and teeth	fiber for regularity

INGREDIENTS

Burgers:

- 3 tablespoons chopped dill
- 2 shallots, chopped
- 2 teaspoons Dijon mustard
- 1 pound skinless center-cut salmon, chopped into ½-inch cubes
- ¼ teaspoon salt
- ¼ teaspoon black pepper
- ⅓ cup panko bread crumbs
- 4 whole grain buns
- 1 tomato, sliced
- 2 cups arugula

Sauce:

- 1 ripe avocado
- ½ cup sour cream
- 1 tablespoon prepared horseradish
- 1 tablespoon lemon juice

DIRECTIONS

- Preheat grill to medium. In a food processor, blend dill, shallots, mustard, half of the salmon, salt, and pepper into a pastry-like puree. Add remaining salmon and breadcrumbs and pulse just until combined. Form into 4 equal-sized patties and brush with oil. Grill 4 minutes per side, or just until cooked through.

- To make the sauce, mash together avocado, sour cream, horseradish, and lemon juice in a bowl.

- Toast buns, cut side down, on the grill about 30 seconds. Place salmon burgers on bun bottoms and add sauce, tomato, arugula, and bun tops.

Per Serving: 545 calories, 32 g protein, 51 g carbohydrates, 25 g fat (6g sat.), 92 mg calcium, 3 mg iron, 92 mcg folate, 10 g fiber, 720 mg sodium

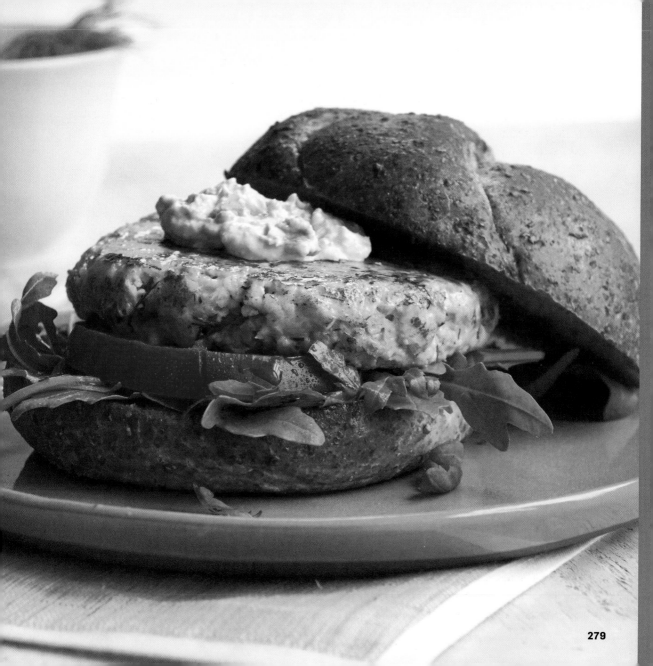

Greek Nachos

Greek yogurt gives the classic Mexican dish a decidedly Mediterranean spin and lets you indulge in cheesy goodness without getting ginormous.

PREP • Active: 15 minutes • Total: 20 minutes • Makes 2 servings

Yogurt	Hummus	Lemon juice	Feta
loaded with calcium for baby's teeth and bones	high quality plant protein for building muscle	vitamin C for baby's growth and morning sickness help	low calorie protein and calcium (make sure it's pasteurized)

INGREDIENTS

- ½ cup nonfat Greek yogurt
- 3 tablespoons fresh lemon juice
- 2 teaspoons plus 2 tablespoons fresh mint, finely chopped
- 1½ teaspoons honey, divided
- 1 small garlic clove, minced
- 4 teaspoons white wine vinegar
- ¼ teaspoon kosher salt
- 1 pint grape tomatoes, diced
- ½ cucumber, diced
- ¼ cup red onion, finely chopped
- ¼ cup Kalamata olives, pitted and chopped
- 1 8-ounce bag plain pita chips
- ⅔ cup prepared hummus
- ½ cup reduced-fat pasteurized feta, divided

DIRECTIONS

- Preheat oven to 350 F. In a small bowl, combine yogurt, 1 tablespoon lemon juice, 2 teaspoons mint, 1 teaspoon honey and garlic. Set aside.

- In a medium bowl, whisk together remaining lemon juice and honey with olive oil, vinegar, and salt. Add tomatoes, cucumber, onion, and olives; toss well.

- Arrange pita chips on an ovenproof platter. Dot with small dollops of hummus; sprinkle with all but 2 tablespoons feta.

- Bake for 5 minutes, then top with dollops of yogurt sauce. Stir tomato misture well and, using a slotted utensil to drain excess liquid, spoon over nachos. Sprinkle with remaining feta and garnish with remaining mint. Serve immediately.

Per Serving: 237 calories, 7 g protein, 27 g carbohydrates, 11 g fat (1g sat.), 91 mg calcium, 1 mg iron, 26 mcg folate, 2 g fiber, 627 mg sodium

Grilled Zucchini Salad with Walnuts, Pomegranates & Mint-Tahini Dressing

This salad can serve as side or entrée; you can add grilled chicken or even steak to boost the staying power. The tahini imparts an earthy, creamy essence and you don't need extra oil because it's high in good fat.

PREP • Active: 30 minutes • Total: 30 minutes • Makes 4 servings

Walnuts	Pomegranate seeds	Tahini
high-quality plant based omega-3s for brain development and protein for building muscle	provide iron—essential for building healthy blood cells—and vitamin C that helps you absorb it	rich in healthy oils essential for development of the placenta, milk glands, and uterus; also a good source of copper and manganese—key to baby's growth

INGREDIENTS

- ½ **cup walnuts, halved**
- 2 **large zucchini, halved crosswise then sliced lengthwise into ¼-inch thick pieces**
- 3 **tablespoons extra virgin olive oil**

Salt and pepper

- ¼ **cup fresh lemon juice**
- 1 **garlic clove, minced**
- 3 **tablespoons fresh mint, finely chopped, divided**
- 2 **tablespoons tahini**
- ¼ **teaspoon chili flakes**
- ½ **cup pomegranate seeds**

DIRECTIONS

- Place walnuts in a small, nonstick pan and toast over medium heat until fragrant; shake the pan frequently and watch closely to prevent burning. Place in a small bowl and set aside.

- Light a grill or heat a grill pan over medium high heat. In a large mixing bowl, toss zucchini with oil and sprinkle with salt and pepper. Grill the zucchini in batches until tender and slightly charred, about 2–3 minutes per side. Remove grilled pieces to a large serving plate and keep warm.

- In a small mixing bowl, whisk lemon juice, garlic, 2 tablespoons mint and, a big pinch of salt. Add tahini and chili flakes, whisk until well combined. Dressing should be easily pourable; if too thick, add a teaspoon or so of water in a slow stream.

- Sprinkle zucchini with walnuts and pomegranate seeds, then drizzle with dressing. Garnish with remaining chopped mint.

Per Serving: 247 calories, 5 g protein, 11 g carbohydrates, 23 g fat (3g sat.), 49 mg calcium, 1 mg iron, 63 mcg folate, 3 g fiber, 52 mg sodium

Roasted Apple–Rosemary Chicken Thighs

That "apple a day" adage is no joke. Eating them keeps blood sugar steady and may even reduce your baby's risk of asthma.

PREP • Active: 15 minutes • Total: 30 minutes • Makes 4 servings

Apples	Chicken	Rosemary
vitamin C, folate; apples eaten during pregnancy may reduce children's asthma risk	lean protein, vitamin B-12 for energy and niacin for brain development	a whiff may improve cognition and memory, also rich in fiber and is an anti-inflammatory

INGREDIENTS

- ½ **pound Granny Smith apples, cored and cubed**
- 1 **pound boneless, skinless chicken thighs, cut into 1-inch-strips**
- 2 **tablespoons white wine**
- 2 **tablespoons olive oil**
- 1½ **teaspoons finely chopped fresh rosemary**
- 2 **garlic cloves, minced**
- ½ **teaspoon kosher salt**
- ½ **teaspoon black pepper**
- 2 **cups cooked brown rice**

DIRECTIONS

- Preheat oven to 400 F. In a large baking dish, combine apples, chicken thighs, wine, olive oil, rosemary, garlic, salt, and pepper. Toss to coat.

- Roast for 20 to 25 minutes or until apples are soft and chicken is cooked through.

- Divide brown rice evenly among 4 plates and top with equal amounts of chicken and apples. Pour pan juices over the top and serve.

Per Serving: 351 calories, 25 g protein, 32 g carbohydrates, 12 g fat (2 g sat.), 2 mg iron, 16 mcg folate, 2 g fiber, 338 mg sodium

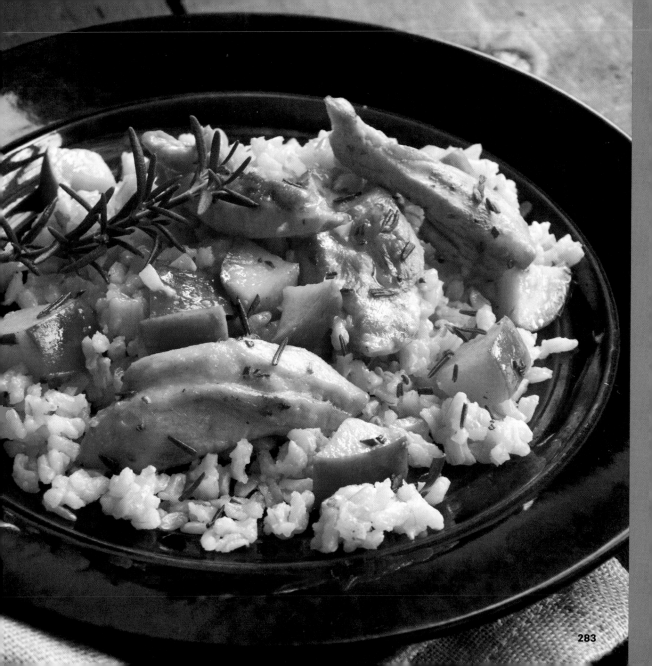

Lime-Glazed Shortbread

These buttery cookies sneak in a little citrus, which can ease nausea,
along with good grain whole wheat, for fiber, antioxidants, and B vitamins.

PREP ● Active: 25 minutes ● Total: 55 minutes ● Makes 30 cookies

Whole wheat	Egg	Olive oil	Lime
B vitamins, iron, and magnesium for building bones	lean protein for muscles	Healthy fat and antioxidants	Eases morning sickness; packed with vitamin C

INGREDIENTS

Cookies:

- **2 cups white whole-wheat flour**
- **½ teaspoon baking soda**
- **¼ teaspoon salt**
- **½ cup turbinado sugar**
- **⅓ cup olive oil**
- **1 large egg, slightly beaten**
- **2 tablespoons honey**
- **2 teaspoons finely grated lime zest**

Glaze:

- **2 cups confectioner's sugar**
- **2 to 3 teaspoons fresh lime juice**
- **½ teaspoon lime zest**

DIRECTIONS

- Preheat oven to 350 F. Line a large baking sheet with parchment paper or silicone liner.

- In a small bowl, combine flour, baking soda, and salt.

- In a large bowl, beat sugar, olive oil, egg, and honey with an electric mixer for 2 minutes. Stir in lime zest and flour mixture until combined (it will be somewhat sticky). On a floured work surface, form dough into a log about 8 inches long and 1½ inches in diameter; wrap in wax paper and refrigerate for 15 minutes or until firm.

- Slice the chilled dough into ¼-inch thick rounds and place on prepared baking sheet. Bake for about 8 minutes or until lightly browned. Let cool 5 minutes on sheet, transfer to a wire rack placed over wax paper, and cool completely.

- Meanwhile, in a small bowl, whisk together confectioner's sugar, lime juice, and zest, adding more juice if necessary to thin the glaze. Drizzle over cookies and let set for 15 minutes.

Per Serving (1 cookie): 73 calories, 1 g protein, 12 g carbohydrates, 3 g fat (0g sat.), 1 mg calcium, 0 mg iron, 1 g fiber, 43 mg sodium

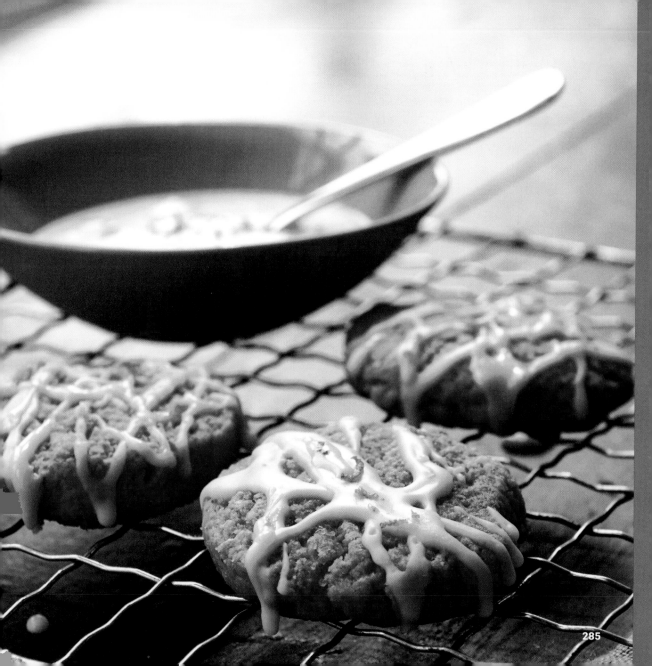

Avocado Chocolate Pudding

Avocados sometimes think they're cream. They can be used to make velvety smoothies and desserts, without the dairy. Avos also are packed with folic acid, which protects against neural tube defects, and healthy omega-3s that promote muscle and brain development.

PREP ● Active: 10 minutes ● Total: 70 minutes ● Makes 3 servings

Avocado	Dates	Cinnamon
Healthy, vegan fats and protein for brain and muscle	high in fiber and iron, and are a rich source of vitamins and minerals.	has been shown to improve blood sugar, so may reduce risk of gestational diabetes.

INGREDIENTS

1 **ripe avocado**

1 **ripe banana**

6 **pitted dates**

¼ **cup unsweetened almond milk**

1 **teaspoon vanilla extract**

¼ **cup cocoa powder**

¼ **teaspoon cinnamon**

Dash of salt

DIRECTIONS

- Blend avocado, banana, almond milk, dates, and vanilla extract in a food processor until smooth.

- Add cocoa powder, cinnamon, and salt. Blend for 1 minute until evenly combined. Refrigerate for 1 hour before serving.

Per Serving: 206 calories, 4 g protein, 30 g carbohydrates, 11 g fat (2 g sat.), 44 mg calcium, 2 mg iron, 67 mcg folate, 9g fiber, 119mg sodium

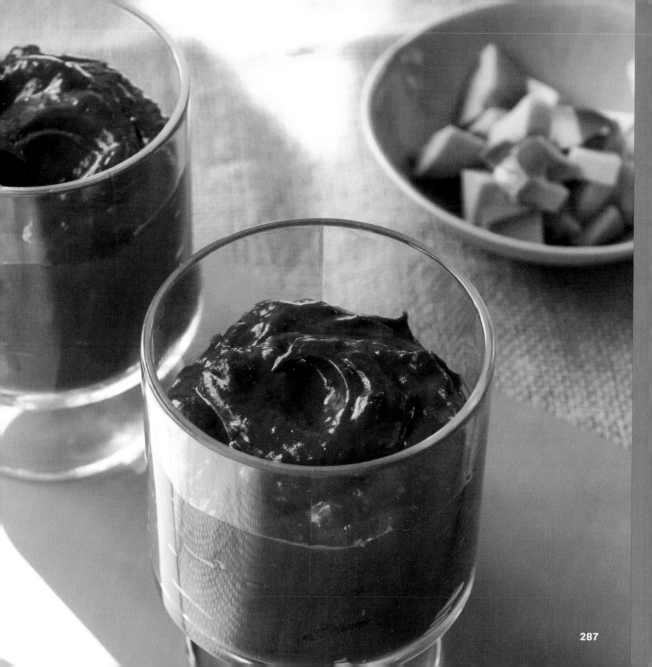

Strawberry Peach Parfaits

Whip up this indulgent parfait, which gives you and your baby fresh-from-the farmers-market peaches and berries (rich sources of fiber and antioxidants) with a splash of cream. The pretty layers will impress, regardless of your pastry skills.

PREP ● Active: 15 minutes ● Total: 15 minutes ● Makes 4 servings

Sour cream and whipped cream
lots of calcium, for bones and teeth

Berries & peaches
pack in fiber and antioxidants for you and plenty of vitamin C for baby, and to help iron absorption

INGREDIENTS

¼ **cup fat-free sour cream**

½ **cup confectioner's sugar, divided**

1 **tablespoon grated orange peel**

3 **tablespoons orange juice**

1½ **cups heavy cream, whipped**

1 **cup raspberries**

3 **cups strawberries**

4 **ripe peaches, cut into ½-inch-thick slices**

DIRECTIONS

● In a bowl, mix sour cream, 6 tablespoons of confectioner's sugar, orange zest, and juice. Fold whipped cream into the mixture.

● Puree the raspberries with remaining sugar in a food processor; fold strawberries into raspberry sauce.

● Divide peaches between 4 glasses. Spoon most of sour cream mixture over each, dividing evenly. Top with the strawberries and a dollop of remaining cream mixture; garnish with strips of orange peel.

Per Serving: 374 calories, 6 g protein, 52 g carbohydrates, 18 g fat (11g sat.), 135 mg calcium, 1 mg iron, 45 mcg folate, 7 g fiber, 54 g sodium

Weeks 14-28

- Breakfast
- Lunch
- Dinner
- Dessert

Second Trimester

It's known as the glow trimester—the second trimester is when you feel like eating, moving, dancing again. And you are busy building that bebe. The dishes in this section are a bit higher in calories, and we've included suggestions for adding the 350 extra you'll need, while still getting the healthy fats, vitamins, and minerals you and your baby need.

Spinach, Herb, & Goat Cheese Fritatta

By using half whole eggs and half egg white, you get the yolks' nutrients—especially choline and omega-3s for baby's brain development—with less cholesterol.

PREP • Active: 20 minutes • Total: 30 minutes • Makes 4 servings

Eggs	Spinach	Parsley
choline, which helps brain cells develop, protects against neural tube defects, and may prevent mental illness	high in calcium and iron	an underrated super food with more nutritional density than kale

INGREDIENTS

- 5 **large eggs**
- 5 **large egg whites**
- 1 **medium leek or small onion**
- 3 **cups baby spinach leaves**
- ½ **cup fresh Italian parsley leaves**
- 40 **chives (about ½ bunch)**
- 1 **tablespoon olive oil**
- ¼ **teaspoon salt**
- ¼ **teaspoon freshly ground black pepper**
- 2 **ounces soft pasteurized goat cheese**

DIRECTIONS

- Preheat the broiler.

- Combine the whole eggs, egg whites, and 2 tablespoons of water in a medium bowl and whisk well.

- If using leek, slice off the dark green top and discard. Slice remaining white and light green parts in half lengthwise and rinse well, then finely chop. Otherwise, dice the onion. Coarsely chop the spinach, parsley, and all but about 8 of the chives.

- Heat the olive oil in a medium cast-iron or nonstick ovenproof skillet over medium heat.

- Add the leek or onion and cook, stirring, until it begins to soften, about 3 minutes. Add the spinach, parsley, chives, salt, and pepper and cook for 1 minute, until spinach just begins to wilt.

- Pour egg mixture over greens in the skillet, covering them evenly. Decrease heat to medium-low and cook until egg mixture has set around the edges but not in the middle, 8 to 10 minutes.

- Distribute the cheese over the eggs in 10 to 12 dollops and scatter the reserved whole chives on top. Place skillet under the broiler about two inches from the heat and broil until surface is set and golden brown, 1 to 2 minutes. Be careful not to overcook or eggs will become tough.

- Cut frittata into 4 wedges and serve immediately.

Per Serving: 204 calories, 16 g protein, 7 g carbohydrates, 13 g fat (5 g sat.), 100 mg calcium, 3 mg iron, 65 mcg folate, 2 g fiber, 393 mg sodium

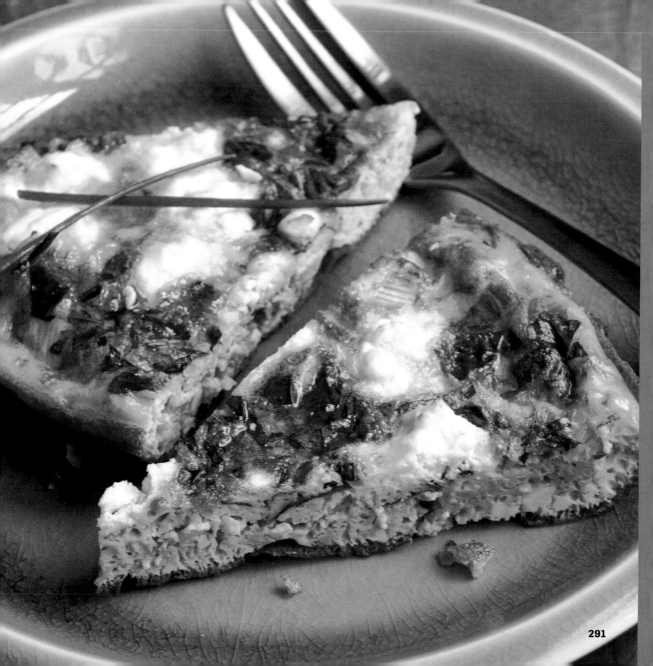

Blueberry Cornmeal Pancakes

Heart-healthy flaxseeds and protein-rich pecans turn these vegan flapjacks into a super stack. A drizzle of organic maple syrup may even boost immunity.

PREP • Active: 20 minutes • Total: 30 minutes • Makes 6 servings

Almond milk	Flaxseed	Pecans	Blueberries
high in calcium for your and baby's bones and teeth	vegan source of omega-3s, high in fiber	high quality vegan fat and protein	vitamin C and antioxidants

INGREDIENTS

- 1½ **cups plain, unsweetened almond milk**
- 1 **tablespoon plus 1 teaspoon fresh lemon juice**
- 2 **tablespoons ground flaxseed**
- ¼ **cup hot water (about 180 F)**
- ¼ **cup canola oil**
- 1½ **cups whole-wheat pastry flour**
- ⅔ **cup cornmeal**
- 2 **tablespoons granulated sugar**
- 1 **teaspoon baking powder**
- ½ **teaspoon salt**
- 2 **cups blueberries, plus 2 cups for topping**
- 1 **cup pecans, toasted and coarsely chopped**
- **Confectioner's sugar (optional)**
- **Organic maple syrup (optional)**

DIRECTIONS

- In a large mixing bowl, whisk together almond milk and lemon juice. Let mixture sit for 5 to 10 minutes to thicken into a buttermilk-like consistency.

- In a small bowl, stir ground flaxseed and hot water together. Allow to sit for 5 to 10 minutes as it thickens.

- Add flaxseed mixture and canola oil to the "buttermilk" and whisk to combine.

- In a medium mixing bowl, stir together the flour, cornmeal, granulated sugar, baking powder, and salt. Then, stir the dry ingredients into the wet until just combined, and then fold in the blueberries. If the batter is too thick to pour, thin it with a little more almond milk.

- Heat a medium cast-iron skillet or nonstick griddle over medium heat. When the pan is hot, brush it with a thin layer of oil. Spoon a scant ¼ cup of batter onto the griddle for each cake. This should spread to form a 4-inch pancake. Cook for 2 minutes, until batter begins to bubble and the bottoms are golden brown. Flip the pancakes and cook until both sides are golden brown. Repeat with remaining batter. Top pancakes with a sprinkle of pecans, additional blueberries, and a dusting of confectioner's sugar, if desired. Finish with organic maple syrup.

Per Serving: 406 calories, 7 g protein, 42 g carbohydrates, 26 g fat (2 g sat.), 255 mg calcium, 2 mg iron, 19 mcg folate, 7 g fiber, 438 mg sodium

Turkey Burger Mediterranean Style

Here, we complement truly lean turkey with a barrage of big flavors—punchy olives, sweet red peppers, a layer of tangy pasteurized feta cheese—that do little to compromise the overall nutritional picture.

PREP • Active: 17 minutes • Total: 17 minutes • Makes 4 servings

Lean turkey	**Pasteurized feta cheese**	**Red peppers**
good source of B vitamins, not to mention protein	did we mention it needs to be pasteurized?	each one filled with vitamin C

INGREDIENTS

- 1 lb lean ground turkey
- Salt and pepper to taste
- ½ teaspoon dried thyme
- ½ cup pasteurized feta
- 2 cups arugula
- 4 whole wheat English muffins, split and lightly toasted
- ½ cup roasted red peppers
- ¼ cup olives, chopped

DIRECTIONS

- Preheat a grill or grill pan. Season turkey with a few big pinches of salt and pepper, plus the dried thyme. Form the meat into four patties, being careful not to overwork the meat (which will cause the proteins to bind, making for a tough burger). Use your thumb to make a small impression in the middle of each patty (as they cook, the middle will swell up; this simple step makes for a more evenly cooked burger).

- Cook over medium-high heat for 4 to 5 minutes on the first side, until lightly charred. Flip and immediately add the cheese to each patty. Cook for another 4 to 5 minutes, until the burgers feel firm and springy to the touch. Remove from the grill.

- Lay the arugula on the bottom of four English muffin halves. Top with the burger, then crown the burger with peppers, olives, and the other half of the English muffin.

Per Serving: 355 calories, 35 g protein, 30 g carbs, 14 g fat (4 g sat.), 2.5 mg iron, 57 mcg folate, 6 g fiber, 760 mg sodium

Chicken Tenders with Peach BBQ Sauce

Tenders cook quickly so you'll spend less time in the heat; you'll also benefit from their payload of protein, a building block for your baby's development.

PREP ● Active: 25 minutes ● Total: 35 minutes ● Makes 6 servings

Peaches	Tomato	Chicken
vitamin C for building connective tissue, folate for NTD protection, and postassium to prevent muscle cramps, fatigue and anxiety	rich in lycopene to protect from cell damage, vitamin C and iron, and folate	lean protein, vitamin B 12; choose organic if possible

INGREDIENTS

- 3 **medium peaches**
- 2 **tablespoons tomato paste**
- 2 **shallots, chopped**
- 2 **cloves garlic, minced**
- 2 **tablespoons cider vinegar**
- 1 **tablespoon brown sugar**
- 1 **tablespoon Worchestershire sauce**
- 1 **teaspoon paprika**
- ½ **teaspoon ground allspice**
- ½ **teaspoon black pepper, divided**
- 1½ **pounds chicken tenders**
- 2 **teaspoons canola oil**

DIRECTIONS

- Slice peaches in half, remove pits, and roughly chop. Place peaches, tomato paste, shallots, garlic, vinegar, brown sugar, Worcestershire sauce, paprika, allspice, ¼ teaspoon each salt, and pepper, and ¼ cup water in a blender or food processor and blend until smooth. Divide peach sauce into two bowls.

- Preheat grill to medium. Brush chicken tenders with oil and season with remaining salt and pepper; grill for 3 minutes, flip, and spread on half of the peach sauce. Continue to grill until inside is no longer pink, 3 to 5 minutes.

- Remove chicken from the grill and brush on the other half of the peach sauce that was not in contact with raw meat. If you like, heat remaining sauce to serve on the side.

Per Serving: 161 calories, 27 g protein, 10 g carbohydrates, 2 g fat (0 g sat.), 12 mg calcium, 1 mg iron, 9 mcg folate, 2 g fiber, 274 mg sodium

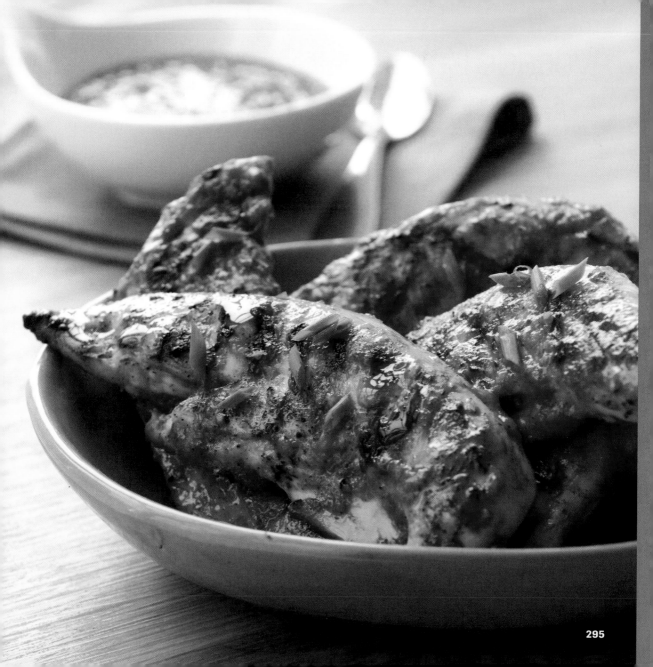

Avocado Crab Salad

Bursting with folate and vitamin B6, avocados nurture your baby's muscle and brain development. Folic acid, of course, protects against neural tube defects such as spina bifida, and the omega-3s in the avocado boost baby's brain development and your mood and skin. Vitamin B6 also helps detoxify the liver.

PREP ● Active: 15 minutes ● Total: 15 minutes ● Makes 4 servings

Avocado	Fennel	Crabmeat
folate for NTD protection, vitamin B6 to form new red blood cells and antibodies, vital to baby's brain and nervous system development.	helps balance hormones, soothe indigestion, and may increase breast milk production.	great source of protein, vitamin D for bone health and choline for brain development, minerals iron, zinc, iodine, copper, and selenium, and omega-3s for protection against depression

INGREDIENTS

- 1 **fennel bulb, thinly sliced**
- ½ **Fuji apple, thinly sliced**
- 2 **cups arugula**
- 1 **ripe avocado, cubed**
- ½ **cup lump crabmeat**
- 2 **tablespoons lemon juice**
- 2 **tablespoons extra virgin olive oil**
- 1 **teaspoon agave nectar**
- 1 **teaspoon dried oregano**
- ¼ **teaspoon sea salt**

DIRECTIONS

- Combine fennel, arugula, and cubed avocado. Add crabmeat and toss. Add apple.

- In a small bowl, whisk together lemon juice, olive oil, agave nectar, oregano, and sea salt. Pour just enough over salt to coat well.

- Toss and serve.

Per Serving: 118 calories, 4 g protein, 14 g carbohydrates, 15 g fat (2 g sat.), 69 mg calcium, 1 mg iron, 74 mcg folate, 6 g fiber, 228 mg sodium

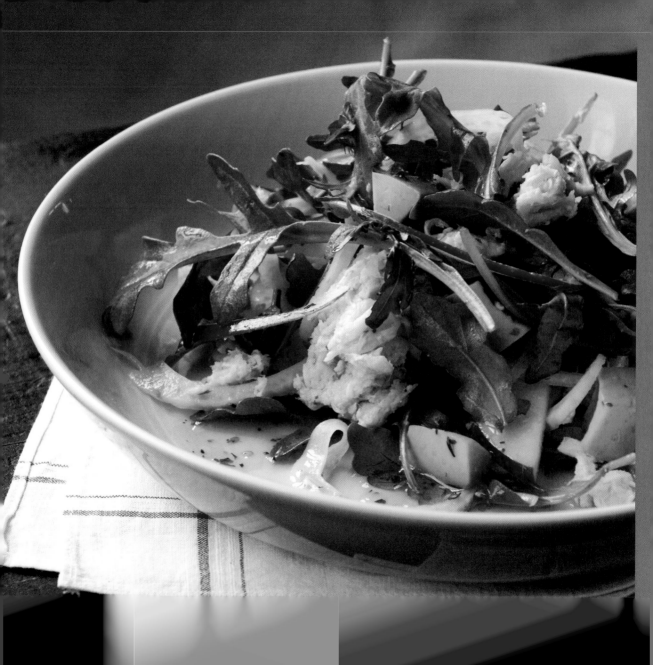

Fennel-Crusted Roasted Chicken
with Smashed Sweet Potatoes

Toasted fennel gives this simple, elegant dish nutty flavor, and the sweet potatoes are loaded with nutrients. Experiment with adding lemon or paprika to the rub, and you can make extra and store in the fridge for all kinds of dishes.

PREP • Active: 15 minutes • Total: 1 hour, 45 minutes • Makes 6 servings

Sweet potatoes	Fennel	Cast iron pan
potassium, essential for baby's growth and prevents leg cramps; also high in vitamin C and iron	a mild remedy for infertility and promotes lactation	boosts iron intake

INGREDIENTS

- 2 **tablespoons fennel seeds, plus 1 teaspoon**
- 1 **stick unsalted butter, plus two tablespoons, room temp**
- **Salt and black pepper**
- 1 **small yellow onion, sliced**
- 1 **4-pound whole fresh chicken**
- 3 **garlic cloves, peeled**
- 3 **medium sweet potatoes**

Per Serving: 669 calories, 39 g protein, 16 g carbohydrates, 49 g fat (21g sat.), 81 mg calcium, 3 mg iron, 22 mcg folate, 3 g fiber, 181 mg sodium

DIRECTIONS

- Preheat oven to 425 F. Toast fennel seeds in a medium cast iron pan over high heat for 3 minutes. Crush in a mortar and pestle (or with the bottom of a smaller pan).

- In a large bowl, combine butter and crushed fennel seeds. Season with salt and freshly ground black pepper. Separate 2 tablespoons of butter mixture and set aside.

- Place sliced onion in a roasting tray. Season chicken cavity with salt and pepper, and place garlic inside. Arrange chicken in roasting tray on top of onions. Using your fingers, separate the skin from the breast and smear some of the fennel butter rub into this pocket. Smear the rest on the outside of the bird, getting into all the gaps between the legs and wings. Season liberally with salt and pepper. Tie the legs with kitchen twine.

- Place tray in the center of the oven and roast for 15 minutes, then reduce heat to 350 F.

- Prepare sweet potatoes: Prick all over with a fork, then place on a small tray in the same oven as the chicken; bake together for 1 hour.

- Remove chicken from oven and let rest for 15 minutes before carving. Remove sweet potatoes from oven and let cool slightly. Cut sweet potatoes open and scoop flesh into a large bowl. Add the reserved compound butter and smash with potato masher. Serve sweet potatoes with chicken.

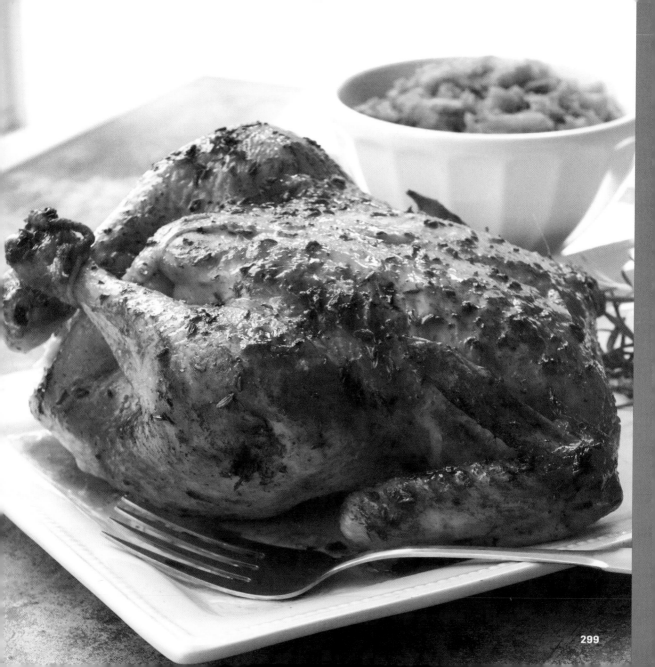

Apple-Carrot Slaw with Toasted Coconut

You can satisfy pregnancy cravings with this slaw made with a combo of sweet, spicy, and crunchy. Apples also are a great source of fiber.

PREP ● Active: 15 minutes ● Total: 15 minutes ● Makes 4 servings

Apples	Olive oil	Coconut
fiber and recent research shows they might reduce risk of asthma	packed with antioxidants and healthy fats; also used to lubricate the perineum to prevent tears and episiotomy during delivery	source of healthy fats, and coconut oil has been shown to ease morning sickness, constipation, and indigestion during pregnancy

INGREDIENTS

- ¼ cup unsweetened coconut
- ½ teaspoon cumin seeds
- 1½ teaspoons lemon juice
- ¼ teaspoon salt
- pinch of cayenne pepper
- 2 tablespoons olive oil
- ½ pound Macoun apples
- ½ pound carrots, grated
- 1 tablespoon chives
- 1 tablespoon flat-leaf parsley, chopped

DIRECTIONS

- Toast coconut in small skillet over medium heat, tossing occasionally, for 3 to 5 minutes. Add cumin and toast 30 seconds longer. Remove from pan and cool completely.

- In a small bowl, prepare dressing: Whisk together lemon juice, salt, cayenne pepper, and olive oil. Set aside.

- Quarter, core, and thinly slice apples. Toss in a large bowl with grated carrots. Add coconut mixture and lemon dressing, then toss in chives and parsley. Toss to coat all and serve immediately.

Per Serving: 155 calories, 1 g protein, 15 g carbohydrates, 11 g fat (4 g sat.), 27 g calcium, 1 mg iron, 15 mcg folate, 4 g fiber, 163 mg sodium

Bejeweled Biscotti

These gorgeous cookies are loaded with fruit and nuts, making them festive and healthful. A whiff of the orange zest can stave off the queasies, and the pistachios and olive oil supply antioxidants.

PREP ● Active: 20 minutes ● Total: 1 hour, 10 minutes ● Makes 30 cookies

Coriander	Cinnamon	Dried fruit
used to boost milk production	helps stabilize blood sugar	packed with antioxidants and vitamin C

INGREDIENTS

- 2 cups whole-wheat flour
- ½ cup almond flour
- 1 teaspoon baking powder
- 1 teaspoon ground coriander
- 1 teaspoon ground cinnamon
- ¼ teaspoon salt
- 2 large eggs, 1 separated
- ¼ cup light olive oil
- ½ cup plus 1 tablespoon turbinado sugar
- 2 teaspoons finely grated orange zest
- ½ cup coarsely chopped dried apricots
- ½ cup coarsely chopped dried cranberries
- ½ cup coarsely chopped unsalted pistachios

DIRECTIONS

- Preheat oven to 350 F. Line a large baking sheet with parchment paper or a silicone liner.

- In a medium bowl, whisk together flours, baking powder, cinnamon, coriander and salt. Set aside.

- In a bowl, beat together 1 whole egg, 1 yolk (reserve egg white), olive oil, and ½ cup sugar with a wooden spoon until smooth. Gradually add the flour mixture until just combined. Stir in orange zest, dried fruit, and pistachios.

- On a floured work surface, form dough into 2 logs about 10 inches long. Place on baking sheet and flatten each log until about 1 inch thick and 2 inches wide. Brush with reserved egg white and sprinkle with reserved tablespoon of sugar.

- Bake for about 30 minutes or until cookies are lightly browned and surfaces begin to crack. Remove from oven and cool for 10 minutes, then place legs onto a cutting board.

- Reduce oven temp to 325 F. When logs are cool enough to handle, cut into ½-inch-thick slices using a serrated knife. Return slices to baking sheet and bake for 10 to 15 minutes longer, depending on desired crispness. Cool completely on a wire rack.

Per Serving: 95 calories, 2 g protein, 13 g carbohydrates, 4 g fat (1g sat.), 13 mg calcium, 2 g fiber, 33 mg sodium

Grilled Fruit Salad with Banana Ice Cream

Grilling fruit supercharges its natural sweetness, making it the star of this dessert. The Harvard Nurses' Study found that eating nuts during pregnancy might prevent kids' nut allergies. And the potassium in bananas helps quell morning sickness and ease leg cramps.

PREP ● Active: 25 minutes ● Total: 30 minutes ● Makes 6 servings

Mangoes
As is the other fruit in this dish, mangoes are rich in fiber to help constipation, and also in folate, vitamins A, C and B6, all vital for you and your baby

Pistachios
may prevent kids' nut allergies, and supply iron, folate, calcium and potassium

INGREDIENTS

- 2 **mangoes, peeled, pitted and cut into 1-inch-thick slices**
- 3 **nectarines, cut in half, pits removed**
- 4 **plums, cut in half, pits removed**
- 2 **teaspoons canola oil**
- 1 **lime, juiced (about 2 tablespoons)**
- ½ **cup dark chocolate chunks**
- ½ **cup pistachios, roughly chopped**
- ⅓ **cup dried coconut flakes**
- 4 **medium frozen bananas, chopped**
- ¼ **cup light coconut milk**
- 2 **teaspoons vanilla extract**

DIRECTIONS

- Preheat grill to medium. Lightly brush cut sides of fresh fruit pieces with oil before placing them on grill grate, cut sides down. Cook until grill marks appear and fruit softens. Remove fruit from grill, let cool, and then chop.

- In a large bowl, toss fruit with lime juice. Stir in chocolate, pistachios, and coconut flakes.

- To make banana ice cream, place frozen bananas, coconut milk and vanilla extract in a food processor or high-powered blender and blend until smooth and creamy. Serve immediately, or place in freezer in an airtight container until ready to use. Before serving, let ice cream sit at room temperature for a few minutes to soften.

- Place fruit salad in bowls, top with banana ice cream, and serve immediately.

Per Serving: 402 calories, 6 g protein, 58 g carbohydrates, 17 g fat (8 g sat.), 36 mg calcium, 1 mg iron, 76 mcg folate, 9 g fiber, 8 mg sodium

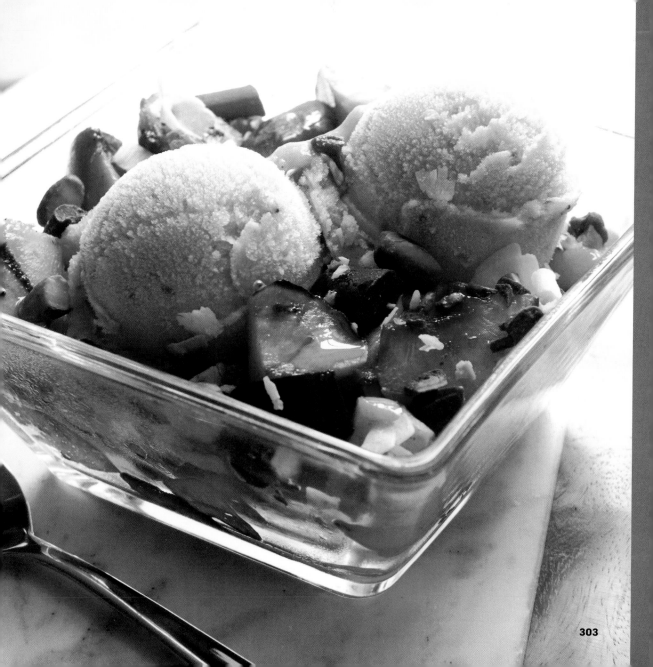

Brown Butter Apple Crumble

Tart Granny Smith apples, butter, sugar, and cinnamon = heaven. And this dessert comes with benefits; apples are full of antioxidants and the spices have anti-inflammatory action as well. Sweet!

PREP ● Active: 15 minutes ● Total: 1 hour ● Makes eight servings

Apples
packed with fiber and disease-fighting antioxidants

Cinnamon
helps regulate blood sugar and ease inflammation

INGREDIENTS

- **4 Granny Smith apples, diced**
- **½ tablespoon lemon juice**
- **1 tablespoon granulated sugar**
- **⅔ cup, plus 1 tablespoon all-purpose flour**
- **¾ cup brown sugar**
- **1 teaspoon cinnamon**
- **¼ teaspoon nutmeg**
- **¼ teaspoon salt**
- **6 tablespoons unsalted butter**

DIRECTIONS

- Preheat oven to 350 F. Combine apples, lemon juice, granulated sugar, and 1 tablespoon flour in a bowl. Pour into 9-inch pie pan.

- In a separate bowl, combine ⅔ cup flour, brown sugar, cinnamon, nutmeg, and salt.

- In a saucepan over medium heat, melt butter, stirring occasionally, until it begins to turn golden, about 10 minutes. Drizzle into flour and spice blend, stirring with a fork until the mixture is crumbly.

- Spread over apples and bake 35 to 40 minutes, until apples are bubbling and topping has browned. Divide into 8 glass dessert cups and serve warm.

Per Serving: 270 calories, 2 g protein, 48 g carbohydrates, 9 g fat (6 g sat.), 35 mg calcium, 1 mg iron, 22 mcg folate, 3 g fiber, 80 mg sodium

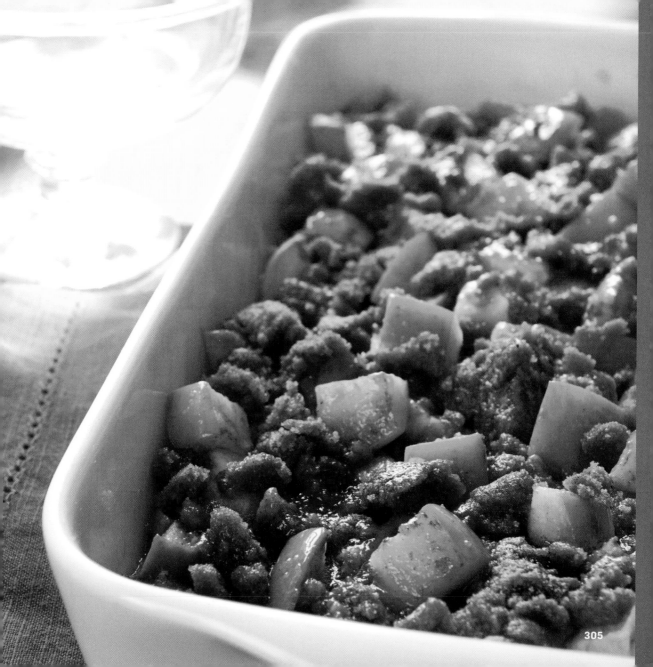

Weeks 28–40

- Breakfast
- Lunch
- Dinner
- Dessert

Third Trimester

You are approaching the home stretch, and when you are in your third trimester, your nutritional needs are very similar to your second; the difference is that your stomach itself is getting squished by your baby, so you might need to split up your meals into smaller portions. For example, eat your salad first, and save your entrée for later.

Oatmeal with Peanut Butter and Banana

Plain oats are too boring to eat on a regular basis, and flavored oats carry a bevy of excess sugars. We solve both problems by using peanut butter and almonds to provide a rich base of healthy fats.

PREP • Active: 10 minutes • Total: 10 minutes • Makes 4 servings

Rolled oats	Peanut Butter	Bananas
packed with fiber, to keep things moving	may prevent peanut allergies in your child	the potassium helps your electrolyte balance, which keeps your fluids right

INGREDIENTS

4½ cups water

2 cups rolled oats

Pinch of salt

2 bananas, sliced

2 tbsp peanut butter

¼ cup chopped almonds

2 tbsp agave syrup

DIRECTIONS

- In a medium saucepan, bring the water to a boil. Turn the heat down to low and add the oatmeal and salt. Cook, stirring occasionally, for about 5 minutes, until the oats are tender and have absorbed most of the liquid.

- Add the bananas, peanut butter, almonds, and agave syrup and stir to incorporate evenly. If the oatmeal is too thick, add a splash of milk.

Per serving: 328 calories, 10 g protein, 52 g carbs, 10 g fat (2 g sat.), 3 mg iron, 37 mcg folate, 7 g fiber, 50 mg sodium

Greens and Grains Scramble

Whether you choose baby kale, spinach, Swiss chard, or all of the above, a fresh mix of greens delivers essential nutrients (calcium plus vitamins A, C, and K) to nourish you and your bambino.

PREP • Active: 25 minutes • Total: 75 minutes • Makes 2 servings

Whole grains	**Dark, leafy greens**	**Eggs**	**Olive oil**
explode with folate , which protects against NTDs	a great source of calcium, especially if you are vegan	protein for muscle development, choline for brain development	healthy fat, rich in antioxidants and anti-inflammatory properties

INGREDIENTS

- 2 **large eggs**
- 1 **tablespoon milk**
- ¼ **teaspoon kosher salt**
- 2 **tablespoons extra virgin olive oil**
- 1 **whole green onion, finely chopped (about 1 tablespoon)**
- 2 **cloves garlic, minced**
- 1 **heaping cup leafy greens**
- ½ **cup cooked whole grains (wheat berries, faro, barley, or millet)**
- 1 **tablespoon fresh chives, chopped**
- **Freshly ground black pepper**
- **Flaky sea salt (such as Maldon)**
- **Crusty bread, toasted English muffins, or warm corn tortillas for serving**

DIRECTIONS

- In a large bowl, whisk together eggs, milk, and kosher salt; set aside. Heat 1 tablespoon of olive oil in a nonstick pan over medium heat. Add the green onion and garlic and sauté until soft, 1 to 2 minutes. Add greens, grains, and remaining 1 tablespoon olive oil and sauté until greens are wilted and grains are warmed, 3 to 5 minutes.

- Decrease heat to low and pour in egg mixture, gently stirring to combine it with the greens and grains. Continue stirring until eggs are softly scrambled, 2 to 3 minutes. Remove from the heat, stir in chives, and season with pepper.

- Serve hot with a sprinkling of sea salt on top and bread, English muffins, or tortillas on the side.

Per Serving: 334 calories, 15 g protein, 15 g carbohydrates, 24 g fat (15g sat.), 125 mg calcium, 2 mg iron, 111 mcg folate, 2 g fiber, 398 mg sodium

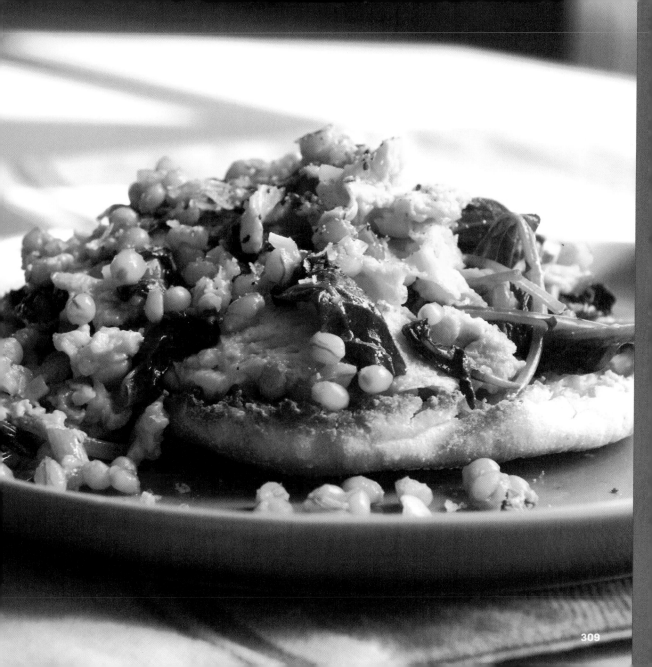

French Toast Fingers

These indulgent sticks are pleasingly sweet but also pack fiber thanks to their whole-wheat base.

PREP ● Active: 40 minutes ● Total: 40 minutes ● Makes 4 servings

Almonds healthy fats and omega 3s	**Whole wheat bread** fiber and folate	**Blueberries** antioxidants and vitamin C

INGREDIENTS

- 1 **cup sliced almonds**
- 3 **cups cornflakes**
- ½ **teaspoon ground cinnamon**
- ½ **teaspoon ground nutmeg**
- ¼ **teaspoon salt**
- 2 **large eggs**
- ¾ **cup low-fat milk**
- 1 **tablespoon pure maple syrup**
- 1 **teaspoon vanilla extract**
- 4 **large slices firm whole-grain bread, each piece cut crosswise to make 5 fingers**
- **Blueberry Maple Sauce (recipe follows) or maple syrup (optional)**

DIRECTIONS

- In a food processor, pulse the almonds until coarsely ground. Add the cornflakes, cinnamon, nutmeg, and salt, then pulse until the cornflakes resemble the texture of oats. Transfer mixture to a shallow bowl.

- In a medium bowl, whisk the eggs, milk, maple syrup, and vanilla until combined.

- Spray a large nonstick skillet or griddle with a cooking spray and preheat over medium heat.

- Working with 1 piece at a time, dip the bread into the egg mixture until completely moistened and coated but not falling apart, about 15 seconds on each side. Coat each stick with the cornflake mixture, gently pressing it into the bread. Place each stick in the skillet and cook over medium-low heat, turning once, until the outside is golden brown and the center is warm, about 6 minutes. Repeat with each stick.

- Serve with Blueberry Maple Sauce.

Per Serving (5 sticks): 283 calories, 11 g protein, 30 g carbohydrates, 15 g fat (2 g sat.), 141 mg calcium, 5 mg iron, 47 mcg folate, 4 g fiber, 351 mg sodium

Blueberry Maple Sauce

INGREDIENTS

- 2 **cups fresh or frozen (unsweetened) blueberries**
- 1 **tablespoon pure maple syrup**
- 1 **tablespoon orange juice**

DIRECTIONS

- In a medium saucepan, combine the blueberries, maple syrup, and orange juice. Bring mixture to a gentle boil. Reduce to medium-low heat and simmer, stirring occasionally, for 2 minutes.

- Transfer the mixture to a blender and blend until almost smooth. Add more maple syrup to taste, depending on the sweetness of the fruit. The sauce may be made up to 4 days in advance and stored in an air-tight container in the fridge.

Per Serving (2 tablespoons): 57 calories, 1 g protein, 14 g carbohydrates, 0 g fat, 10 mg calcium, 0 mg iron, 6 mcg folate, 2 g fiber, 1 mg sodium

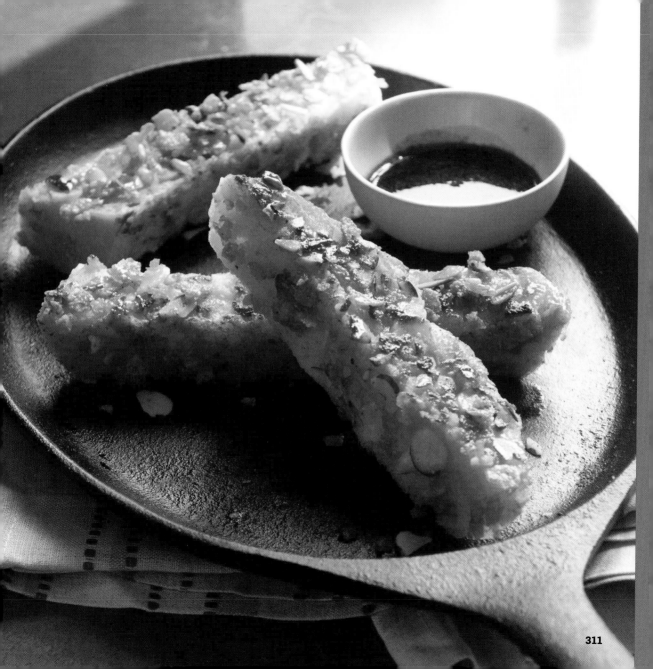

Potato Kale Salad with Yogurt Dressing

Kale brings vitamins A, C, and K to the carb-bomb that is traditional potato salad. Beyond bolstering your immunity and digestive health, the probiotics in yogurt can slash the risk for preeclampsia by about 20 percent, according to a study in the *American Journal of Epidemiology*. Tip: to avoid a soggy salad, make sure the potatoes have cooled before mixing with yogurt dressing, and cut your spuds into equal chunks so they cook evenly.

PREP ● Active: 15 minutes ● Total: 80 minutes ● Makes 6 servings

Kale
rich source of vitamin K, which is essential for blood clotting and to prevent newborn hemorrhaging

Yogurt
provides probiotics for gut health and strong immunity

INGREDIENTS

- 2 **pounds small red-skinned potatoes, quartered**
- 2 **teaspoons grapeseed or canola oil**
- 6 **cups chopped kale**
- ⅓ **cup chopped chives**
- ¼ **cup low-fat plain yogurt**
- ½ **cup oil-packed sun-dried tomatoes, chopped**
- 2 **teaspoons Dijon mustard**
- 1 **teaspoon lemon zest**
- ½ **lemon, juiced (about 1 ½ tablespoons)**
- ¼ **teaspoon salt**
- ¼ **teaspoon black pepper**

DIRECTIONS

- Preheat oven to 400 F. Toss potatoes with oil and spread on a baking sheet. Bake for 35 minutes or until tender. Spread the kale over the potatoes, return to oven, turn off the heat and let rest 5 minutes. (The kale will wilt in the residual heat.) Remove vegetables from oven and let cool for about 15 minutes.

- In a medium bowl, whisk together yogurt, tomatoes, chives, mustard, lemon zest, lemon juice, salt, and pepper. Toss yogurt mixture with vegetables until everything is coated. Serve immediately.

Per Serving: 295 calories, 10 g protein, 42 g carbohydrates, 11 g fat (1 g sat.), 214 mg calcium, 42 mg iron, 56 mcg folate, 6 g fiber, 206 mg sodium

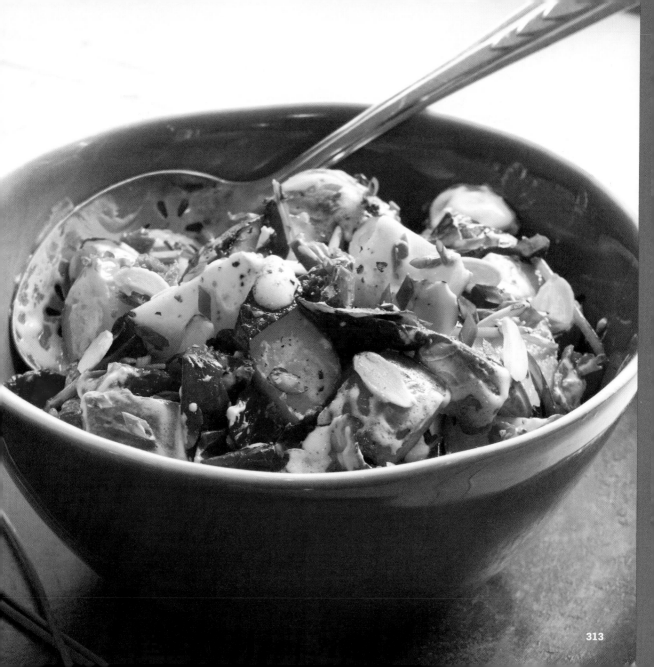

Avocado Enchilada

Yes, avocado mashed with jalapeno, garlic, and lime juice is delicious, but take your adventurous palate further with this simple Mexican dish.
Postnatal bonus: Can be frozen and stored for quick dinners after the baby comes.

PREP • Active: 15 minutes • Total: 35 minutes • Makes 3 servings

Chicken
rich source of amino acids for building baby's muscle, also provides vitamin E, selenium, thiamine, and niacin to boost metabolism and energy.

Yogurt
probiotics for overall and digestive health; low fat, vegetarian protein source

INGREDIENTS

- 1 **cup low-sodium enchilada sauce (divided)**
- 1 **ripe avocado**
- ¼ **cup plain nonfat Greek yogurt**
- ¼ **teaspoon minced garlic**
- 1 **tablespoon ground cumin**
- 2 **teaspoons hot sauce**
- ¼ **fresh tomato salsa**
- ¼ **cup white onion, chopped**
- 6 **low-carb tortillas**
- 8 **ounces cooked chicken, cubed (divided)**

DIRECTIONS

- Preheat oven to 350 F. Coat an 8-by-8-inch pan with cooking spray, then pour in ¼ cup enchilada sauce.

- Mash avocado with yogurt, garlic, cumin, hot sauce, and salsa.

- Saute onion. Layer each of the tortillas with the avocado mixture, chicken, and onion. Roll up and place side by side in pan. Drizzle with ¾ cup enchilada sauce; bake for 20 minutes.

Per Serving: 118 calories, 4 g protein, 14 g carbohydrates, 15 g fat (2 g sat.), 50 mg calcium, 2 mg iron, 60 mcg folate, 5 g fiber, 10 mg sodium

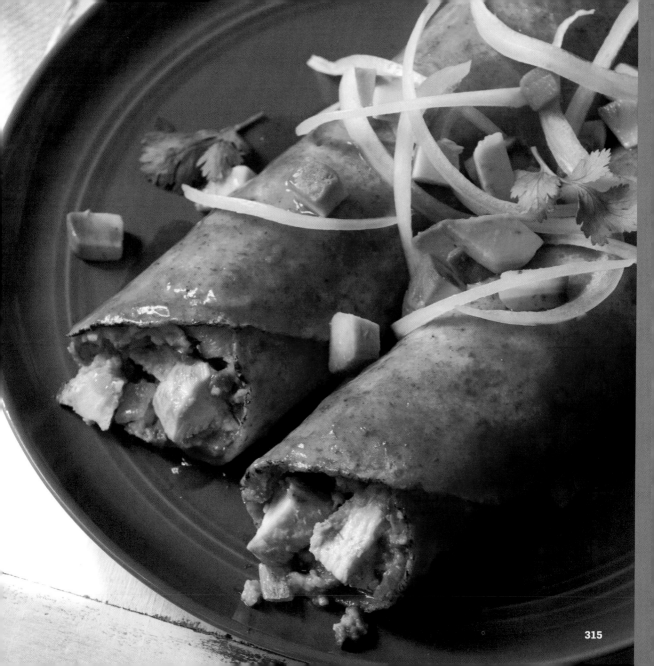

Steamed Snapper with Fresh Ginger & Lime

This is straightforward, simple good food with very pregnancy-friendly ingredients such as ginger and lime. Snapper is on the mercury-safe list; use this method to cook other fish, too. And the leftovers taste great, so perfect for post-natal stocking up.

PREP • Active: 30 minutes • Total: 45 minutes • Makes 4 servings

Snapper	Grapefruit and lime	Ginger
Mercury-safe omega-3s for your baby's brain development and your peace of mind; fish oils also impart anti-inflammatory properties	loaded with vitamin C for baby's immunity and muscle development	eases nausea and indigestion, helps body absorb nutrients, balances blood glucose levels, pain relief

INGREDIENTS

- 6 **scallions, green parts trimmed**
- 1 **lime, juiced (about 2 tablespoons)**
- 2 **tablespoons grapefruit juice**
- 2 **tablespoons peanut oil**
- **Salt and freshly ground pepper**
- 4 **6-ounce boneless/skinless snapper filets**
- 1 **1-inch piece of fresh ginger, peeled and julienned**
- 2 **garlic cloves, peeled and thinly sliced**
- 1 **lime, thinly sliced**
- 1 **cup cilantro leaves, for garnish**
- 2 **scallions, thinly sliced on the bias for garnish**
- 2 **cups steamed jasmine rice, for serving**

DIRECTIONS

- Preheat oven to 450 F. Cut six scallions in half lengthwise to create 12 equal-length batons, each about 4–5 inches long (they should be the same length as your filets).

- Prepare marinade: In a small mixing bowl, whisk together lime juice, grapefruit juice, peanut oil, and a healthy pinch of salt and pepper. Cut 4 squares of parchment paper (each about 17 inches long) and fold in half so they have a crease down the middle.

- Working with one portion at a time, place 3 scallion batons side by side in the center of each parchment square just to one side of the crease. Place 1 fish filet on top, then top with a little julienned ginger and sliced garlic. Add about 1 tablespoon of the marinade over each filet and cover with 3 lime slices.

- Fold parchment over fish, then make small overlapping folds along the perimeter to secure the pouch. At the corners, you can make a deeper fold to end up with a half-moon shaped pocket. Place pouches on a roasting tray and bake in the oven until the parchment has puffed up and browned slightly, about 12 minutes.

- Serve individual pouches on plates and cut open, being careful of the steam that is released. Garnish with cilantro and scallion. Serve with steamed rice.

Per Serving: 344 calories, 37 g protein, 28 g carbohydrates, 10 g fat (2 g sat.), 60 mg calcium, 2 mg iron, 77 mcg folate, 3 g fiber, 10 mg sodium

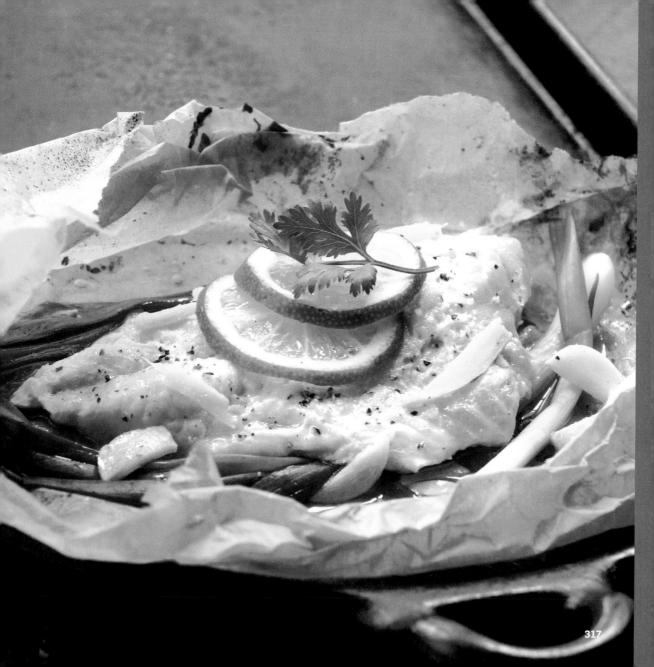

Hearty Beef Stew

Loaded with iron (from the beef) and vitamins (thanks to the vegetables), this dish will satisfy your and your baby's nutrient needs now, and will deliver a substantial quick meal you can just pop in the microwave, if you like. The slow cooker method makes it beautifully simple.

DIRECTIONS

- Combine 3 pounds of chunked beef (chuck or round), 1 can of diced tomatoes, and 1 can of reduced-sodium beef broth. Add vegetables (e.g. frozen peas, zucchini, and baby carrots), garlic, oregano, paprika, and rosemary to taste. Cook in a slow cooker on low for 7 hours. Freeze in tightly-sealed containers.

Unfried Stir Fry

Simple nourishing ingredients such as broccoli and snow peas make an Asian-inspired dish nourish now and even better later as flavors blend.

DIRECTIONS

- Layer cooked brown rice or quinoa, bite-sized baked tofu or tempeh, sliced raw veggies (like broccoli, snow peas and asparagus), and your favorite sauce (try mixing peanut butter with soy sauce, in a small glass container) and store in fridge or freeze. To reheat or defrost the meal and simultaneously steam the vegetables, add a tablespoon of water and microwave in 90-second intervals, stirring between, until heated.

PB & J Fingerprint Cookies

A twist on a childhood fave, this cookie packs cramp-nixing potassium

An oatmeal base and raspberry jam sing along with wholesome, creamy peanut butter; even just one will satisfy sweet, savory, and crunchy cravings. And the banana is packed with potassium, which prevents leg cramps.

PREP ● Active: 15 minutes ● Total: 25 minutes ● Makes 24 cookies

Bananas potassium for leg-cramp relief	**Oats** folate, iron, B vitamins, and fiber (very important in your third trimester)

INGREDIENTS

- 1½ **cups whole-wheat pastry flour**
- ¼ **cup old-fashioned rolled oats**
- 1 **teaspoon baking powder**
- ¼ **teaspoon salt**
- ½ **cup natural creamy peanut butter (no salt added)**
- 1 **medium banana, mashed**
- ½ **cup light brown sugar**
- 1 **large egg white**
- ¼ **cup all-fruit raspberry jam**

DIRECTIONS

- Preheat oven to 350 F. Line a large baking sheet with parchment paper or silicone liner.

- In a medium bowl, whisk together flour, oats, baking powder, and salt. Set aside.

- In a large bowl, combine peanut butter, banana, sugar, and egg white with a wooden spoon or electric mixer set to medium, until smooth. Add the flour mixture gradually and beat until combined.

- Form dough into 1-inch balls, place on baking sheet 1 inch apart, and make an indentation in the center of each cookie with your thumb. Fill each with about ½ teaspoon of jam.

- Bake for about 10 minutes or until cookies are lightly browned and jam is just starting to bubble. Let cool 5 minutes on the sheet, then transfer to a wire rack and cool completely.

Per Serving (1 cookie): 90 calories, 3 g protein, 14 g carbohydrates, 3 g fat (0 g sat.), 13 mg calcium, 1 mg iron, 3 g fiber, 38 mg sodium

Almond Crisps

The nuts in this super simple and satisfying cookie help foster your baby's bone development and are easy to digest for you, a blessed relief in the third trimester.

PREP ● Active: 15 minutes ● Total 30 minutes ● Makes 20 cookies

INGREDIENTS

- 3 **large egg whites, at room temp**
- ½ **cup superfine sugar**
- 1 **teaspoon pure vanilla extract**
- 3 **cups (12 ounces) sliced almonds with skins, lightly toasted**

DIRECTIONS

- Position racks in the center and top third of the oven and preheat to 350 F. Line 2 baking sheets with parchment paper.
- Whisk egg whites in a medium bowl until foamy, then mix in sugar and vanilla. Gently fold almonds into mixture.
- Place a 2½-inch round cookie cutter on top of prepared baking sheet. Fill with 2 tablespoons of cookie mixture and press down to flatten. Remove cutter and shape remaining crisps, spacing them 1 inch apart.
- Bake for 8 minutes, then switch the trays' positions and cook for 5 minutes more or until golden. Remove from oven and cool on a wire rack.

Per Serving: 120 calories, 4 g protein, 9 g carbohydrates, 8 g fat (1 g sat.), 50 mg calcium, 1 mg iron, 1 mcg folate, 2 g fiber, 5 mg sodium

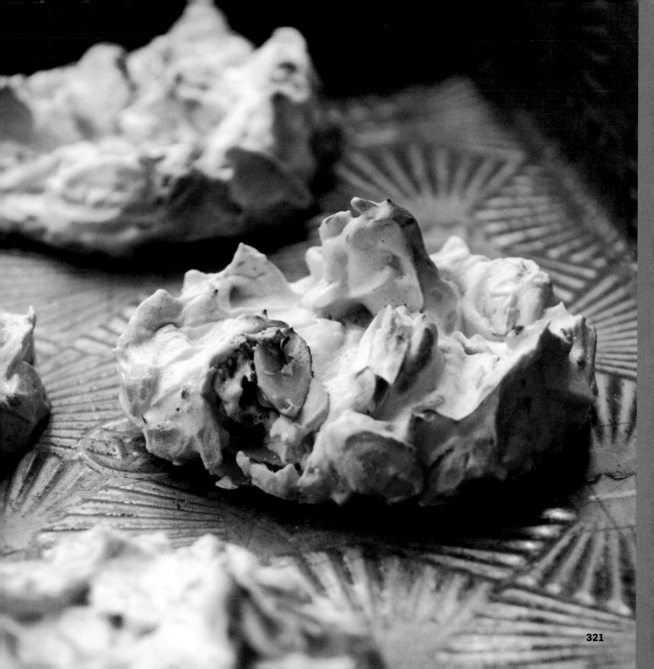

Caramel Apple Bread Pudding

Bread puddings are super easy and can be assembled ahead of time; then throw in the oven as you start eating. It'll be ready when you're finished with your main course. The leftovers taste great, too. Apples are good for you and your baby, and the cinnamon and sugar will make you and everyone around you happy.

PREP ● Active: 1 hour ● Total: 1 hour, 10 minutes ● Makes 4 servings

Milk	Cinnamon
easy to digest source of calcium, it also may help you sleep	blood sugar regulation, possibly protecting against gestational diabetes

INGREDIENTS

- ½ **pound brioche, cut into 1-inch pieces (6 cups)**
- 2½ **tablespoons unsalted butter**
- 1 **large Granny Smith apple, peeled, cored and cut into ½-inch pieces**
- ½ **cup sugar**
- ¼ **teaspoon cinnamon**
- ⅛ **cup apple cider**
- 2 **large eggs, beaten**
- 1½ **cups milk**
- ½ **vanilla bean, split**
- ¼ **cup dulce de leche**
- **Vanilla ice cream (optional)**

DIRECTIONS

- Preheat oven to 350 F. Spread the brioche on a rimmed baking sheet. Toast for about 15 minutes, stirring once or twice until lightly golden.

- Meanwhile, in a large skillet, melt butter; reserve 1 ½ tablespoons melted butter in a small bowl. Add apples and ⅛ cup of the sugar to the skillet and cook over moderate heat, stirring occasionally, until the apples are golden and softened, about 15 minutes. Stir in cinnamon and apple cider. Cook until sauce is syrupy, about 2 minutes.

- In a large bowl, whisk eggs with milk and remaining sugar to create the custard. Scrape in seeds from the vanilla bean. Add brioche and apples and toss until evenly coated. Let stand for 5 minutes.

- Brush an 8-by-8-inch baking dish with ½ tablespoon of melted butter. Add bread pudding and drizzle remaining tablespoon of melted butter and dulce de leche on top. Bake until custard is set and the top is golden, about 40 minutes. Let cool slightly. Serve with ice cream and more dulce de leche, if desired.

Per Serving: 256 calories, 6 g protein, 38 g carbohydrates, 10 g fat (5 g sat.), 92 mg calcium, 9 mcg folate, 1 mg iron, 1 g fiber, 183 mg sodium

Virgin Salty Dog

Here's how to not feel left out at a party: Sip on this fizzy, festive warm-weather mocktail.

PREP • Makes 1 drink

INGREDIENTS

2½ ounces grapefruit juice

¾ ounce grenadine syrup

½ ounce verjus (available online and in specialty stores)

¼ ounce lime juice

Pinch of salt

Tonic water

Maraschino cherry

DIRECTIONS

- Shake first 5 ingredients together in a shaker with ice.
- Pour into a highball glass.
- Top with tonic water.
- Garnish with a maraschino cherry

Mexican Hot Chocolate

For a cold-weather treat with a kick, cozy up to some sweet and creamy. Not that you need an excuse, but drinking milk may lead to taller children, says a study in the *European Journal for Clinical Nutrition*.

INGREDIENTS

1 cup nonfat milk

1 cinnamon stick

Pinch ground cayenne pepper

1 tablespoon unsweetened cocoa powder

2 teaspoons granulated sugar

½ teaspoon vanilla extract

Pinch ground cinnamon

DIRECTIONS

- Heat the milk, cinnamon stick, and cayenne pepper in a small saucepan over medium heat until simmering. Turn off burner and let stand for 5 minutes. Discard cinnamon stick.
- Whisk in the cocoa powder and sugar and warm over low heat just until hot. Remove from stove, whisk in vanilla. Sprinkle with a dusting of ground cinnamon.

Index

Recipes